D0549577

Shaomin Yan

Myocyte Nuclear Chamges in End-Stage Cardiomyopathies

Shaomin Yan

Myocyte Nuclear Chamges in End-Stage Cardiomyopathies

Quantitative Diagnostic Pathology

LAP LAMBERT Academic Publishing

Impressum / Imprint
Bibliografische Information der Deutschen Nationalbibliothek: Die Deutsche Nationalbibliothek verzeichnet diese Publikation in der Deutschen Nationalbibliografie; detaillierte bibliografische Daten sind im Internet über http://dnb.d-nb.de abrufbar.
Alle in diesem Buch genannten Marken und Produktnamen unterliegen warenzeichen-, marken- oder patentrechtlichem Schutz bzw. sind Warenzeichen oder eingetragene Warenzeichen der jeweiligen Inhaber. Die Wiedergabe von Marken, Produktnamen, Gebrauchsnamen, Handelsnamen, Warenbezeichnungen u.s.w. in diesem Werk berechtigt auch ohne besondere Kennzeichnung nicht zu der Annahme, dass solche Namen im Sinne der Warenzeichen- und Markenschutzgesetzgebung als frei zu betrachten wären und daher von jedermann benutzt werden dürften.

Bibliographic information published by the Deutsche Nationalbibliothek: The Deutsche Nationalbibliothek lists this publication in the Deutsche Nationalbibliografie; detailed bibliographic data are available in the Internet at http://dnb.d-nb.de.
Any brand names and product names mentioned in this book are subject to trademark, brand or patent protection and are trademarks or registered trademarks of their respective holders. The use of brand names, product names, common names, trade names, product descriptions etc. even without a particular marking in this works is in no way to be construed to mean that such names may be regarded as unrestricted in respect of trademark and brand protection legislation and could thus be used by anyone.

Coverbild / Cover image: www.ingimage.com

Verlag / Publisher:
LAP LAMBERT Academic Publishing
ist ein Imprint der / is a trademark of
AV Akademikerverlag GmbH & Co. KG
Heinrich-Böcking-Str. 6-8, 66121 Saarbrücken, Deutschland / Germany
Email: info@lap-publishing.com

Herstellung: siehe letzte Seite /
Printed at: see last page
ISBN: 978-3-659-30800-0

Zugl. / Approved by: Udine, University of Udine, 1999

University of Udine

Myocyte Nuclear Chamges
in End-Stage Cardiomyopathies

Ph.D.- Dissertation in Quantitative Diagnostic
Pathology
Shao-Min Yan

Supervisor
Prof. Carlo Alberto Beltrami

Defendence of this dissertaion was taken place in
Febrary 26^{th,} 1999
University of Siena, Siena, Italy

This dissertaion was updated in October, 2012

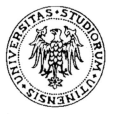

1997/98

This dissertation is dedicated to my beloved father Daguang Yan who died in the earthqueke occurred in Tangshan, China, on July 28, 1976.

Table of Contents

1. SUMMARIES 1

   1.1. Summary in English...1

   1.2. Summary in Italian..6

2. INTRODUCTION 11

   2.1. End-stage cardiomyopathies 11

   2.2. DNA content of myocytes 14

   2.3. Nuclear area of myocytes 17

   2.4. Nuclear mitoses of myocytes..19

   2.5. DNA ploidy patterns of myocytes 20

   2.6. Chromatin bridges..22

   2.7. Aims of the study 24

3. MATERIALS and METHODS 25

   3.1. Determination of DNA ploidy ranges......................................25

   3.2. Estimation of post-mortem changes in DNA content.................26

   3.3. Patient population 26

   3.4. Preparation of myocardial cells 29

   3.5. Image cytometric measurement 29

   3.6. Confocal microscopic assessment 30

   3.7. Statistical analysis...31

4. RESULTS...33

   4.1. DNA ploidy ranges of myocytes 33

   4.2. Post-mortem changes in DNA content 38

   4.3. Anatomical parameters 43

   4.4. Number of nuclei per myocyte 43

   4.5. DNA content of myocytes 46

      4.5.1. DNA content per nucleus 46

      4.5.2. DNA content per cell...51

   4.6. Sum of intermediate ploidies 52

   4.7. Total ploidy index...56

   4.8. Nuclear area of myocardial cells 58

4.8.1. Average nuclear area 58

4.8.2. Coefficient of variation in average nuclear area 61

4.8.3. Nuclear area of myocytes in different DNA ploidy classes 62

4.9. Nuclear mitosis of myocytes...66

4.10. Variety of nuclear DNA ploidy patterns of cardiomyocytes................68

4.10.1. Nuclear DNA ploidy patterns of cardiomyocytes 68

4.10.2. Myocytes with nuclei in different DNA ploidies 72

4.10.3. Myocytes with nuclei in different intermediate ploidies............73

4.11. Myocytes with chromatin bridge and extension..................................74

5. DISCUSSION 77

5.1. DNA ploidy ranges of cardiomyocytes 77

5.2. Post-mortem changes in DNA content 79

5.3. Multinucleation and cardiomyopathies..80

5.4. Polyploidization and cardiomyopathies..82

5.5. Intermediate ploidies and cardiomyopathies 86

5.6. Total ploidy index and cardiomyopathies...88

5.7. Nuclear area and cardiomyopathies..91

5.7.1. Myocyte growth and cardiomyopathies 92

5.7.2. Interstitial cell growth and cardiomyopathies 94

5.8. Myocyte mitosis and cardiomyopathies 96

5.9. Nuclear DNA ploidy patterns of cardiomyocytes 98

5.9.1. Variety of nuclear DNA ploidy patterns in cardiomyocytes.........98

5.9.2. Heterogeneity of nuclear DNA ploidy patterns in multinucleated myocytes100

5.10. Chromatin bridges and cardiomyopathies 101

6. ACKNOWLEDGEMENTS 106

7. REFFERENCES..107

8. ABBREVIATIONS..126

1. SUMMARIES

1.1. Summary in English

Aim of the study

By means of image cytometric and confocal microscopic analyses, quantitative investigations are performed on myocardial cells from adult human hearts. The purposes of this study focus on myocyte nuclear changes in end-stage idiopathic dilated, ischemic and transplanted cardiomyopathies, in order to obtain more details of the following issues:

- DNA ploidy ranges of cardiomyocytes
- post-mortem changes in DNA content of myocardial cells
- degree of polyploidization and multinucleation of cardiomyocytes
- nuclear area of interstitial cells and myocytes
- nuclear DNA ploidy patterns of cardiomyocytes
- myocyte mitoses
- myocytes with chromatin bridge and extension.

Materials and methods

- DNA ploidy ranges of myocytes were evaluated in 74 explanted hearts at biopsy. The ranges of diploidy were calculated by two ways: the mean ± 10% and the mean ± 3SD of integrated optical density (IOD) of interstitial cells. The differences of DNA ploidy ranges between two calculated methods were compared according to the sum of ploidy peaks (SPP) and the sum of intermediate ploidies (SIP).
- Post-mortem changes in DNA content were assessed in 7 bioptic hearts with respect to the fixative time of 1, 8, 16, 24, 36, 48, 72 and 96 hours after cardiac

explantation, prior to the fixation, the tissue samples were stored at 4°C and room temperature.

- Cytometric analysis was performed on 36 autoptic hearts (13 control and 23 transplanted) and on 67 bioptic hearts (37 were idiopathic dilated cardiomyopathy and 30 were ischemic cardiomyopathy). Tissue samples were obtained from the mid section of the lateral wall of left and right ventricles. Myocardial cells were dissociated by 50% KOH and stained by Feulgen reaction. 100 fibroblasts and 200 myocytes were measured in each ventricle. Nuclear number, area, DNA content and DNA ploidy patterns were determined.

- The confocal microscopic observation was performed on 86 hearts (13 control, 25 idiopathic dilated, 25 ischemic and 23 transplanted). Two different sections were selected from the lateral wall of the left ventricle. Nuclear mitosis, chromatin bridges and extensions were observed on YOYO–1 iodide ($\lambda = 488$) stained slides. Myocytes and non-myocytes were distinguished by looking for sarcoplasmic α–sarcomeric actin ($\lambda = 568$). The total of 10000 myocytes was observed in each ventricle.

Results

- The range of DNA ploidies varied according to the different calculating methods. The sum of ploidy peaks of myocytes decreased by 9%, whereas the sum of intermediate ploidies of myocytes increased by 70% calculated by the mean ± 10% as compared to that of calculating it by the mean ± 3SD of IOD of interstitial cells ($p < 0.001$).

- When tissue samples were stored at room temperature, the IOD decreased by 13% at 96 hours after cardiac explantation; the coefficient of variation of IOD increased by 1.1-fold and 1.6-fold at 72 and 96 hours respectively after cardiac explantation; the sum of intermediate ploidies increased about 3 times and 5 times at 72 and 96 hours respectively after cardiac explantation. However, no significant changes in nuclear DNA content were found even at 96 hours after cardiac explantation, when tissue samples were stored at 4°C.

- The cardiomyopathic hearts were characterised by a decrease in mononucleated myocytes and by an increase in binucleated and multinucleated myocytes in both ventricles. The degree of multinucleation appeared striking in dilated hearts and moderate in ischemic hearts.

- A significant decrease in diploid myocytes was found in the cardiomyopathic hearts, meanwhile myocytes with DNA content higher than 4c increased. These features were present in a similar way biventricularly. The increase in the total ploidy index was about 70% and 60% in dilated and ischemic hearts respectively compared to that of control hearts. The most prominent characteristic in the myopathy after cardiac transplantation was a 4-fold increase in the sum of intermediate ploidies. Moreover, when the donor age was smaller than 30 years or the age difference between the recipient and the donor was larger than 25 years, the sum of intermediate ploidies increased about 1-fold, whereas the total ploidy index decreased by 22%.

- The nuclear area of interstitial cells increased about 30% in cardiomyopathic hearts. Augmentation of average nuclear area of myocytes was 1.5-fold, 1.3-fold and 37% in the dilated, ischemic and transplanted groups, respectively. Furthermore, the nuclear area of myocytes enlarged as the augmentation of nuclear DNA content. The relative nuclear areas of myocytes can be presented as:

$$2c : 4c : 8c : 16c : 32c : 64c = 1 : 1.68 : 2.73 : 4.27 : 7.25 : 9.18.$$

- The cardiomyopathic hearts revealed a high occurrence of myocyte mitoses. Average nuclear mitosis of myocytes increased by 6-fold in dilated and ischemic cardiomyopathic hearts. Nuclear mitoses of myocytes appeared prominent in cardiac allografts, especially in the patients who died within six months after transplantation (a 64–fold increase). By contrast, myocyte mitosis represented a declining frequency after six months of cardiac transplantation.

3

- Twelve nuclear DNA ploidy patterns were found in mononucleated myocytes (from subdiploidy to 64c including intermediate ploidies). 59, 114 and 146 nuclear DNA ploidy patterns were found in binucleated, trinucleated, and tetranucleated myocytes, respectively. Myocytes with 5 nuclei were occasionally seen and 20 nuclear DNA ploidy patterns were found in these myocytes. The percentages of myocytes with nuclei in different DNA ploidies increased significantly in cardiomyopathic circumstances.

- In comparison to the control group, the myocytes with chromatin bridge and/or extension increased 25.4-fold, 6.5-fold and 10.7-fold in dilated, ischemic and transplanted hearts, respectively.

Conclusions

- The accuracy of myocyte DNA ploidy ranges is affected not only by the mean value of the integrated optical density (IOD) but also by the coefficient of variation of IOD. Therefore, the mean $\pm$ 3SD of IOD from interstitial cells is preferable for calculating the DNA ploidy ranges of myocytes.

- The post-mortem changes in DNA content of myocytes are not found within 48 hours after death.

- The changes in DNA content of myocytes show two completely different aspects in cardiomyopathic hearts: (i) an increase in the degree of multinucleation and polyploidization, which is prominent in idiopathic dilated hearts, medium in ischemic hearts and limited in transplanted hearts; (ii) an increase in subdiploidy and intermediate ploidies, which relates mainly to myocyte injury induced by apoptosis and necrosis. Both myocyte growth and myocyte injury alter the cardiac function and contribute to adaptation or failure of the heart.

- The increase in nuclear size follows either one of two different processes: the first does not involve an increase in DNA content, whereas the second is concomitant with an increment in DNA content. In the first instance, the enlargement of nuclear size is limited. In the second way, augmentation of nuclear size can become very

4

impressive. Enlargement of nuclear area of myocytes represents a complex process, including simple nuclear hypertrophy, polyploidization and multinucleation. The main pattern of nuclear growth of interstitial cells is nuclear hypertrophy without an increase in DNA content.

- The quantitative measurements indicate that nuclear mitoses of myocytes appear unequivocally in control adult human hearts and increase in pathological hearts. This phenomenon is predominant in transplanted hearts, but the frequency of myocyte mitosis decreases sharply after six months of cardiac transplantation.

- The present investigation demonstrates the variety and the heterogeneity of nuclear DNA ploidy patterns of cardiomyocytes. The cardiomyopathic hearts are characterized by the increase in myocytes with nuclei in different intermediate ploidies and in myocytes with chromatin bridge and/or extension. These findings suggest that the chromosomal aberrartion may be one of the reasons for myocyte dysfunction and myocyte death leading to cardiac deterioration.

Key words: cardiomyopathy, chromatin bridge, DNA content, DNA ploidy patterns, image cytometry, mitosis, nuclear area

1.2. Summary in Italian

Scopo dello studio

Molti studi sono stati eseguiti su cellule miocardiche di cuore umano adulto utilizzando valutazioni quantitative con metodi di analisi di citometria d'immagine e di microscopia confocale. Lo scopo dell'attuale lavoro mira ad ottenere più dettagli sui seguenti parametri e sui loro cambiamenti in condizioni patologiche come la cardiopatia idiopatica dilatativa, la cardiopatia ischemica e i cuori post-trapianto cardiaco ortotopico:

- la distribuzione della ploidia del DNA nei miociti
- il cambiamento post-mortem del contenuto del DNA dei miociti
- il grado di poliploidizzazione e di multinucleazione dei miociti
- l'area nucleare delle cellule interstiziali e dei miociti
- modelli nucleari di ploidia dei miociti
- mitosi dei miociti
- miociti con ponti ed estensioni cromatiniche

Materiali e metodi

- La distribuzione della ploidia del DNA nei miociti è stata valutata su sezioni istologiche di 74 cuori espiantati. Il valore delle cellule diploidi è stato calcolato considerando sia la media della densità ottica integrata (IOD) $\pm$ 3SD delle cellule interstiziali sia la media $\pm$ 10% del valore medio della densità ottica integrata (IOD) sempre delle cellule interstiziali. La differenza del valore tra i due metodi è stata comparata secondo la somma dei picchi di ploidia (SPP) e la somma delle ploidie intermedie (SIP).
- Le variazioni del contenuto del DNA dovute ad artefatti post-mortem sono state valutate utilizzando 7 biopsie di cuori espiantati variando il tempo tra il prelievo e

la fissazione da 1, 8, 16, 24, 36, 48, 72 a 96 ore dopo l'espianto mantenendo i prelievi rispettivamente a 4°C e a 20°C.

• Le analisi di citometria d'immagine sono state eseguite su 36 cuori autoptici (13 cuori provenivano dall'archivio autoptico e appartenevano a pazienti deceduti per cause non cardiache e furono considerati cuori controllo e 23 cuori provenivano da pazienti deceduti in tempi diversi dopo trapianto cardiaco ortotopico) e su 67 cuori espiantati (37 per cardiomiopatia dilatativa idiopatica e 30 per cardiomiopatia ischemica). I prelievi sono stati eseguiti sulla parete laterale del ventricolo destro e sinistro, due centimetri sotto il piano valvolare. I miociti sono stati isolati dopo incubazione con 50% KOH. Le sospensioni con i miociti sono state strisciate su vetrini, colorate con il metodo di Feulgen e analizzate con analizzatore di immagini IBAS2000 (Kontron). Per ogni ventricolo di tutti i cuori sono stati esaminati 100 fibroblasti e 200 miociti. In ogni cuore sono stati valutati: numero di nuclei per miocita, area nucleare, contenuto del DNA per nucleo e modelli nucleare di ploidia dei miociti.

• La presenza di mitosi, ponti ed estensioni cromatiniche nelle cellule miocitarie è stata valutata al microscopio confocale su 86 cuori (13 cuori controllo, 25 cuori espiantati per cardiopatia dilatativa idiopatica, 25 cuori espiantati per cardiopatia ischemica e 23 cuori di pazienti deceduti dopo trapianto cardiaco ortotopico). I prelivi della parete libera del ventricolo sinistro sono stati fissati in formalina e inclusi in paraffina. Sono state eseguite sezioni di 5 micron e colorate con un metodo stechiometrico per la valutazione del DNA nucleare (YOYO-1; $\lambda = 488$) e con l'actina α-sarcomerica sarcoplasmica ($\lambda = 568$) per distinguere le cellule miocitarie dalle interstiziali. Queste sezioni sono state osservate al microscopio confocale (Leica, Germany) per l'evidenziazione delle figure mitotiche, ponti ed estensioni cromatiniche esaminando 10000 miociti in ciascun ventricolo.

Risultati

- La distribuzione della ploidia del DNA varia secondo differenti metodi di calcolo. La somma dei picchi di ploidia dei miociti diminusce del 9%, rispetto alla somma delle ploidie intermedie dei miociti; esse aumenta del 70% calcolando la media ± 10% della media della IOD delle cellule interstiziali come comparato a quella del calcolo secondo la media ± 3SD della IOD delle cellule interstiziali (p < 0.001).

- I cuori espiantati se conservati a temperatura ambiente in assenza di fissativo mostrano variazioni della IOD dovute ad artefatti. Infatti i valori di IOD diminuiscono del 13% dopo 96 ore dal prelievo senza fissazione; e il coefficiente di variazione della IOD aumenta di 1,1-volte a 72 ore e 1,6-volte a 96 ore; la somma delle ploidie intermedie aumenta di circa 3 volte e 5 volte a 72 e 96 ore. Tuttavia, quando i campioni sono conservati a +4°C le alterazioni del contenuto del DNA nucleare non sono significative anche a 96 ore dal prelievo senza fissazione.

- I cuori cardiomiopatici sono caratterizzati da una diminuzione nei miociti mononucleati e da un aumento dei miociti binucleati e multinucleati in entrambi i ventricoli. Il grado di multinucleazione appare più evidente in cuori affetti da cardiopatia dilatativa idiopatica rispetto ai cuori affetti cardiopatia ischemica.

- Una diminuzione significativa dei miociti diploidi è presente nei cuori cardiopatici, con aumento dei miociti con DNA superiore a 4c. Queste variazioni sono simili in entrambi i ventricoli. L'aumento nell' indice totale di ploidia (TPI) è circa del 70% e 60% nei cuori affetti da cardiopatia dilatativa idiopatica ed ischemica rispetto ai cuori controllo. I cuori di pazienti deceduti dopo trapianto cardiaco ortotopico sono caratterizzati da un aumento di circa 4-volte della somma delle ploidie intermedie. Quando l'età del donatore è inferiore a 30 anni oppure quando la differenza dell'età tra il ricevente ed il donatore è maggiore di 25 anni, la somma delle ploidie intermedie aumenta di circa 1-volta, l'indice totale di ploidia diminuisce del 22%.

- L'area nucleare delle cellule interstiziali aumenta di circa il 30% nei cuori cardiopatici. Nelle cardiopatie dilatative idiopatiche, ischemiche e post-trapianto cardiaco l'aumento dell'area nucleare dei miociti è di 1,45-volte, 1,3-volte e 37%

rispettivamente. L'area nucleare dei miociti aumenta con l'aumento del contenuto del DNA. La relativa area nucleare dei miociti può essere presentata come:

2c : 4c : 8c : 16c : 32c : 64c = 1 : 1,65 : 2,75 : 4,60 : 7,25 : 9,18.

- Le figure mitotiche dei miociti aumentano nei cuori cardiopatici. Le mitosi miocitarie aumentano di 6-volte nei cuori affetti da cardiomiopatia dilatativa idiopatica e post-ischemica. Le figure mitotiche sono ancora più numerose nei cuori di pazienti deceduti dopo trapianto cardiaco soprattutto se deceduti entro sei mesi dal trapianto con un aumento di 64-volte.

- Dodici modelli nucleari di ploidia sono stati individuati in miociti mononucleati (dalla subdiploidia a 64c compreso ploidie intermedie). 59, 114 e 146 modelli nucleari di ploidia sono stati individuati in miociti rispettivamente binucleati, trinucleati e tetranucleati. Miociti con 5 nuclei sono stati occasionalmente visti e 20 modelli nucleari di ploidia sono stati individuati in questi miociti. La percentuale dei miociti con nuclei in ploidie differenti aumenta significativamente nei cuori cardiomiopatici.

- Rispetto ai cuori controllo, i miociti con ponti cromatinici e/o estensioni cromatiniche aumentano di 25,4-volte, 6,5-volte e 10,7-volte rispettivamente nei cuori affetti da cardiomiopatia dilatativa idiopatica, ischemica e post-trapianto.

Conclusioni

- La precisione della valutazione della distribuzione della ploidia del DNA nei miociti è condizionata non solo dalla media della densità ottica integrata (IOD) ma anche dal coefficiente di variazione della IOD. Quindi, la media ± 3SD della IOD è utile per calcolare la distribuzione della ploidia del DNA nei miociti.

- Il contenuto del DNA dei miociti non varia entro 48 ore post-mortem.

- Le variazioni del contenuto del DNA dei miociti mostrano due aspetti completamente differenti nei cuori cardiomiopatici: (i) un aumento delle cellule multinucleate e un aumento della poliploidizzazione, che si rileva preminente nei cuori dilatativi idiopatici, medio nei cuori ischemici e limitato nei cuori post-trapianto; (ii) un aumento dei miociti nella subdploidia e nelle ploidie intermedie, indice di un danneggiamento cardiaco indotto principalmente da apoptosi e necrosi. La proliferazione miocitaria e la perdita dei miociti sotto forma di apoptosi o di necrosi contribuiscono entrambi al rimodellamento cardiaco sia nelle cardiopatie, sia nel cuore dopo trapianto cardiaco e influenzano la funzionalità cardiaca contribuendo all'adattamento o all'insufficenza del cuore.

- L' aumento delle dimensioni nucleari segue uno dei due differenti processi: il primo non coinvolge l' aumento del contenuto del DNA, mentre il secondo è correlato con un incremento del contenuto del DNA. Nella prima circostanza, l'allargamento delle dimensioni nucleari è limitato. Nel secondo caso, l'aumento delle dimensioni nucleari può diventare impressionante. L'aumento dell'area nucleare dei miociti rappresenta un complicato processo comprendente ipertrofia nucleare semplice, poliploidizzazione e multinucleazione. L'aumento dell'area nucleare nelle cellule interstiziali è dovuto a ipertrofia nucleare senza aumento del contenuto del DNA.

- La ricerca delle figure mitotiche nei cuori umani conferma la presenza di mitosi miocitare nei cuori controllo ed un loro aumento nei cuori patologici. Questo fenomeno è ancora più accentuato nei cuori dopo trapianto cardiaco soprattutto entro i sei mesi dal trapianto.

- Il presente studio dimostra la varietà e la eterogenità dei modelli nucleari di ploidia di cardiomiociti. I cuori cardiomiopatici sono caratterizzati da un aumento dei miociti con nuclei in ploidie intermedie differenti e dei miociti con ponti cromatinici e/o estensioni cromatiniche. Queste osservazioni suggeriscono che l'aberrazione dei cromosomi potrebbero essere una ragione della disfunzione del miocita e della sua morte portando alla insufficienza cardiaca.

2. INTRODUCTION

2.1. End-stage cardiomyopathies

Cardiac transplantation is the most effective method for treatment of patients with end-stage heart diseases (Pepper *et al.*, 1995). The main indications for heart transplantation are idiopathic dilated cardiomyopathy and ischemic cardiomyopathy. Idiopathic dilated cardiomyopathy defines a pathological condition of the heart characterised by cardiomegaly and ventricular dilation (Lakdawala *et al.*, 2012). Ischemic cardiomyopathy is an anatomical condition initiated by primary events in the coronary circulation. The chronic ischemic cardiomyopathy takes the form of a dilated ischemic myopathy with multiple focal sites of myocardial damage in the ventricular wall (Anversa *et al.*, 1993; Ohara and Little, 2010). In the terminal stage, both of them are characterised by decompensated eccentric left ventricular hypertrophy, myocardial damage with segmental fibrosis, replacement fibrosis and diffuse interstitial fibrosis, significant amount of myocyte loss and reactive hypertrophy of the remaining viable cells (Anversa *et al.*, 1985, 1986). Myocardial scarring, reactive growth processes in myocytes and architectural rearrangement of the muscle compartment of the myocardium all contribute to the ventricular dilation and to the progressive deterioration of cardiac pump function in both these diseases (Beltrami *et al.*, 1994, 1995).

However, it is still difficult to understand the structural basis of heart failure. Hypertrophy and ventricular dilation are apparent, but routine histological observations on tissue sections display normal myocardium, except of little damage represented by focal areas of reparative and interstitial fibrosis (Roberts, 1976; Schuster and Bulkley, 1980; Pantely and Bristow, 1984; Warnes and Roberts, 1984; Buja and Willerson, 1987; Arbustini *et al.*, 1991; Anversa *et al.*, 1992; Beltrami *et*

11

al., 1995; Li *et al.*, 2004). Although the accumulation of collagen is significant in ischemic cardiomyopathy, the amount of intact myocardium exceeds the muscle mass presented in control hearts. The reactive hypertrophy of viable myocytes compensates for the loss of injured tissue (Beltrami *et al.*, 1994).

Changes in the hypertrophied myocardium include expression of fetal protein (Nadal-Ginard and Mahdavi, 1989), mechanical properties of the muscle (Gwathmey *et al.*, 1978, 1990, 1993; Morgan, 1991), composition of the myocyte cytoplasm (Schaper *et al.*, 1991), vascular supply (Rakusan *et al.*, 1992), myosin isozymes (Lowes *et al.*, 1997; Nakao *et al.*, 1997), ventricular geometry and structure (Jugdutt 2012) and so on. Nevertheless, animal experiments indicate that these defects evolve the cardiomyopathies in the early stage (Page, 1978; Anversa *et al.*, 1986, 1993; Capasso *et al.*, 1993; Li *et al.*, 1995, 1997; Liao *et al.*, 1996; Nichtova *et al.*, 2012). The pathogenic mechanisms responsible for the transition to cardiac dysfunction and clinical heart failure are not well understood.

The myopathy that develops following cardiac transplantation is characterised by rejection and remodelling of myocardium. The phenomenon of rejection leads to multiple focal sites of myocyte necrosis across the ventricular wall and coronary vascular disease (Pomerance and Stovin, 1985; Johnson *et al.*, 1989; Rowan and Billingham, 1990; Winters, 1991; Graham, 1992; Tazelaar and Edwands, 1992; Symmans *et al.*, 1994). Necrosis is due to the liberation by the cytotoxic lymphocytes of lytic granules containing a pore-forming protein and enzymes. Cytolysin and serine esterases damage membranes and provoke death of the target cell by osmotic lysis (Suitters *et al.*, 1990; Carlquist *et al.*, 1993; Smith and Ortaldo, 1993). On the other hand, the transplanted heart has to adapt to the increased functional demand associated with anatomical variables of the host, such as an increase in ventricular loading. Therefore, reactive growth may be initiated in the myocardium including genetic expression, DNA synthesis and cellular hyperplasia in myocytic and non-myocytic populations (McMahon and Ratliff, 1990; Di Loreto *et al.*, 1995; Beltrami *et al.*, 1997a).

12

o

A relevant characteristic of pathological hearts is the death of myocytes (Anversa *et al.*, 1997; MacLellan and Schneider, 1997). Historically, there are 3 types of cell death: apoptosis, autophagy and necrosis (Nishida and Otsu, 2008). Although it is well known that necrosis is the main form of myocyte death in myocardium, recent studies have demonstrated that apoptosis occurs in myocardial cells (Masri and Chandrashekhar, 2008). Apoptotic myocyte death has been found in physiological development (Kajstura *et al.*, 1995; Takeda *et al.*, 1996) and in different pathological situations, such as ageing (Kajstura *et al.*, 1996b), congenital heart defects (James *et al.*, 1996; Mallat *et al.*, 1996), end-stage heart failure (Narula *et al.*, 1996; Sharov *et al.*, 1996; Olivetti *et al.*, 1997), hypoxia (Tanaka *et al.*, 1994; Long *et al.*, 1997), ischemic and reperfusion (Gottlieb *et al.*, 1994; Buerke *et al.*, 1995), mechanical stretch (Cheng *et al.*, 1996), myocarditis (Kawano *et al.*, 1994), myocardial infarction (Itoh *et al.*, 1995; Bardales *et al.*, 1996; Kajstura *et al.*, 1996a; Olivetti *et al.*, 1996b), pressure overload cardiac hypertrophy (Teiger *et al.*, 1996), transplanted hearts (Szabolcs *et al.*, 1996; Demetris *et al.*, 1997; Laguens *et al.*, 1997; White *et al.*, 1997) and ventricular pacing (Liu *et al.*, 1995). Thus myocytes can undergo cell death by different mechanisms and the type and magnitude of cell death may differ in various disease circumstances.

Moreover, the affective pathways have been studied in order to understand the translation of mechanical signals into molecular events (Simpson, 1989; Chien *et al.*, 1991; Parker and Schneider, 1991; Anversa *et al.*, 1996a, 1996b, 1998; Wagner and Siddiqui, 2009). The stimuli generated by hemodynamic overloads can lead to an increase in cell size and cell number, i.e., myocyte hypertrophy and myocyte proliferation. However, the information available is limited, especially in human hearts. There is the necessity of further study to understand the transition from normal to abnormal ventricular function and the progression to intractable congestive heart failure.

2.2. DNA content of myocytes

An increase in nuclear DNA content of myocytes in human hearts was first observed by Sandritter and Scomazzoni (1964). Subsequently, Adler and Sandritter (1971) published a paper showing that the DNA content of hypertrophied hearts was increased as a result of the polyploidization of cardiomyocytes. Ebert and Pfitzer (1977) presented a few cases of adult human hearts. The polyploidy was presented in those cases in which scars of the hearts were very old (one to nine years). Two years later, Kazanteva and Babaev (1979) presented a cytophotometric study on ischemic hearts showing an increase in the number of nuclei, in the degree of their ploidy and their correlation with the myocardial mass.

Since 1983, investigations concerning DNA content of myocytes have been increasing. Martynova *et al.* (1983) examined nuclei of myocytes in normal and hypertrophied human heart atrium. The cytophotometric DNA measurements demonstrated the up to 93% occurrence of polyploid nuclei even in myocytes of normal atrium. Myocytes of hypertrophied atrium contained nuclei of higher ploidy degrees. Oberpriller *et al.* (1983) studied the changes in DNA content, number of nuclei and cellular dimensions of young rat atrial myocytes in response to left coronary artery ligation. The results showed that the major responses of atrial myocytes to ventricular infarction were binucleation and a significant increase in DNA ploidy compared to those of sham or control animals. In the same year, Rosenberg and Pfitzer (1983) published their results, in which the great variation in nuclear DNA ploidy of heart muscles persisted in elderly patients. The percentage of nuclei with more than 2c DNA content in both ventricles was correlated with the degree of coronary stenosis and in the right ventricle with the presence and severity of pulmonary emphysema. Using a cytofluorometric nuclear DNA-determination in infant, adolescent, adult and ageing human hearts, Takamatsu *et al.* (1983) concluded that physiological polyploidization progresses in proportion to the increase in the heart weight. Rakusan and Korecky (1985) estimated the regression of cardiomegaly

14

induced by banding the abdominal aorta in new-born rats. In the hearts of banded rats, significantly higher concentrations of RNA and hydroxyproline were found together with decreased concentrations of DNA. However, the total DNA content increased as well as the amount of DNA contributed by muscle cell nuclei. In addition, the percentage of multinucleated myocytes was higher in the hearts from experimental animals. By using quantitative histochemical method, Adler (1986) compared the changes in hypertrophied hearts without and with insufficiency. The results showed that the total DNA content was significantly decreased in insufficient hearts as compared to that of non-insufficient ones. Soon after, Antipanova *et al.* (1987) studied the nuclear DNA content of ventricular, atrial and atrioventricular node myocytes from normal and hypertrophied human hearts. They found a distinct degree of polyploidization and a correlation between DNA content and the number of sex chromatin bodies of myocyte nuclei in different heart compartments. Frenzel *et al.* (1988) studied the regression of cardiac hypertrophy in rat heart after swimming training. At the end of the training period, the heart weight had increased by 65%. A decline in the DNA content by 27% as well as a decrease in the volume density of the interstitial space by 14% and in the number of interstitial cell nuclei by 32% against controls, were explained by a 30% increase in the width of myofibres. In the same year, Vasil'eva and Aref'eva (1988) showed the ratio in the DNA content and protein mass of human cardiomyocytes. DNA level ratio in a number of myocytes of different ploidy were 2 : 4 : 8 : 16 : 32; the same ratio for total protein content was 2 : 3.5 : 6 : 11.4 : 25.5.

In 1990, Rumyantsev *et al.* assessed DNA and sex chromatin content in nuclei of conductive system and working myocytes of normal and hypertrophied human hearts. Myocytes of highly hypertrophied atria contained nuclei of considerably higher ploidy level than those of normal atria. The percentage of binucleated cells showed a 4-fold increase in hypertrophied atria compared with normal ones. The total area of nucleoli per nucleus was proportional to the degree of ploidy. Also, the number of sex chromatin bodies was correlated with ploidy level. By means of cytofluorimetric

15

determination, Luciani *et al.* (1991) studied the nuclear DNA content of myocytes in different sites of the left free ventricular wall in five hearts affected by dilated myocardiopathy. All of the different sites revealed diploid and tetraploid nuclear content. Variable was the presence of octaploid peak: specifically 40% in the external third, 47% in the medium third and 73% in the inner third. Hexadecaploid peak was revealed only twice and exactly in one medium third and in one inner third. These data, even if quite preliminary, suggested the presence of an increasing gradient of ploidization from the external toward the inner part of the left ventricular wall. In 1992, Zerbini *et al.* reported a case of an 8-day-old full-term male infant who had a sudden death. At autopsy was found an enlarged, well-formed heart with biventricular myocardial hyperplasia. DNA ploidy was evaluated by image analysis and showed an abnormal histogram with multiple peaks (2N, 4N and 6N). In the same year, Erokhina *et al.* (1992) evaluated the ultrastructure and biosynthetic activity of polyploid atrial myocytes in patients with mitral valve disease. Polyploid hypertrophied myocytes showed predominant in all the biopsies. The highest extent of cell ploidy was in patients belong to functional class IV according to the classification of New York Heart Association (NYHA); in these cases 72% to 98% of cells had nuclei with 8c and more DNA content. Also in 1992, Kellerman *et al.* determined the nuclear number and DNA content in rat cardiac myocytes from different models of cardiac hypertrophy.

It must be mentioned that two scientific research groups have done a lot of studies on DNA content of myocytes. They are Dr Vliegen with co-workers in the Netherlands and Dr Brodsky with his colleagues in Russia. Using flow cytometry, Vliegen *et al.* evaluated the changes in DNA content of myocytes in normal and hypertrophied hearts (van der Laarse *et al.*, 1987, 1989a, 1989b; Vliegen *et al.*, 1987, 1991). Also, they compared the different responses of cellular DNA content to cardiac hypertrophy in human and rat heart myocytes (Vliegen *et al.*, 1990). From 1980, Brodsky *et al.* have published several articles showing their studies on DNA content of cardiomyocytes. Using image cytometry, they analysed the phenomena of

16

polyploidization and multinucleation of myocytes in animals (Brodsky *et al.,* 1980, 1985, 1986, 1988) and in humans (Brodsky *et al.,* 1993, 1994). Especially, their studies indicated the variability of cardiomyocyte ploidy in normal human hearts (Brodsky *et al.,* 1991).

All of the studies mentioned above show that cardiomyocytes are polyploid and multinucleated population. The degree of polyploidization and multinucleation varies in physiological and pathological conditions. However, some of aspects on this field are yet lack of perfect. The biggest problem probably is that the results of myocyte DNA content were obtained from autopsy human hearts. Although about 25 years ago Adler and Costabel (1975) concluded that no post-mortem changes in DNA content occur even 72 hours after death, a doubt for the statement persists. This is not surprising, considering the variable degree of protein autolysis which may occur rapidly post-mortem. Histones, in particular, are rapidly affected. This may have a main effect on DNA hydrolysis and lead to major and unpredictable errors in the stoichiometry. Thus, it is pressing to do detailed works in order to resolve this problem. Taking the polyploidization of myocyte nuclei into account, few articles deal with the methodological details, such as the determination of the DNA ploidy ranges, intermediate ploidies and so on. Considering the clinical significance, DNA content of myocytes varies so much in normal and pathological states and some reports are contrary. All of these stimulate our interests to do further studies.

2.3. Nuclear area of myocytes

Nuclear size is an objective criterion for analysing various neoplastic tissue lesions. Only a few studies were performed on nuclear size of myocytes. Gerdes *et al.* (1991) examined the changes in nuclear volume and DNA content of cardiac myocytes isolated from weaning, adult and old rats. The results revealed that nuclear volume increased by 79% from weaning to adult. The nuclear length was extended, whereas the nuclear width was unchanged. Nuclear volume was stable from adult to old. In all three rat groups, approximately 98% of myocytes from the left ventricle contained a diploid DNA content. The remainder of nuclei was tetraploid. The degree of polyploidy increased slightly, but significantly, in right ventricular myocytes from old rats. They concluded that the nuclear volume of rat cardiac myocytes increased significantly during normal physiological growth (from weaning to adult), but the rate of nuclear growth was less than that of cell volume. The increase in nuclear size from weaning to adult was not due to an increase in DNA content.

Subsequently, another study was performed to establish whether the nuclear enlargement is also a marker for cellular hypertrophy (Gerdes *et al.*, 1994). Using isolated myocytes, they examined the growth of cardiac myocyte nuclei during cellular hypertrophy in rats with aortocaval fistulas or left ventricular myocardial infarction. The nuclear volume of right ventricular myocytes increased by 24, 55 and 56% in one week, one month and five months after aortocaval fistula surgery, respectively. Increased length, rather than width, accounted for most of the nuclear growth. Nuclear hypertrophy was associated with a progressive increase in cell volume at each time point (34, 88 and 118%). Adaptive growth of left ventricular myocytes followed the same trend, though the extent of cellular and nuclear hypertrophy was reduced. One month after producing a myocardial infarction, there was an increase in nuclear volume (18%) and nuclear length (11%) in right ventricular myocytes, but no changes in the surviving left ventricular myocytes. The cellular volume increased in both right and left ventricles (72 and 18%). Thus, the nuclear size increased as myocytes enlarged, though at a slower rate. Since the nuclear DNA content did not increase in rat with aortocaval fistulas or myocardial infarctions, the increase in nuclear volume was associated with cellular enlargement rather than increased polyploidy.

In 1995, Matturri *et al.* performed morphometric and densitometric approach in hypertrophic cardiomyopathy. Their results showed that the increase in nuclear area and DNA content suggested hyperplasia. The nuclear length and density of myocytes have been evaluated in ischemic cardiomyopathy, dilated cardiomyopathy and right

18

ventricular dysplasia using an image analyzer (Beltrami *et al.*, 1996). Until now, no work has been conducted with respect to the relationship between nuclear size and DNA ploidy classes in human myocardial cells.

2.4. Nuclear mitoses of myocytes

For more than sixty years persists a matter of controversy, which is whether ventricular myocytes retain the capacity to re-enter the cell cycle and proliferate in the adult human heart. As early as 1925, Karsner *et al.* published a paper. They informed that mitotic figures in myocyte nuclei were unable to be detected in histological sections of hypertrophied hearts. Thus, it is a general belief that ventricle muscle cells lose the capacity to proliferate soon after birth (Kranz *et al.*, 1975; Brodsky *et al.*, 1980; Schneider 1986; Ueno 1988; Chien 1991; Cheng *et al.*, 1995). Adult myocytes are terminally differentiated cells and cellular hypertrophy is the only way of growth (Rakusan, 1984).

Conversely, quantitative studies in the failed human hearts challenge this concept. Linzbach concluded that myocyte cellular hyperplasia contributes significantly to myocardial growth in the markedly enlarged decompensated left ventricle (Linzbach, 1960). Subsequently, several works have been done in this field and similar results were obtained (Astorri *et al.*, 1971, 1977; Grajek *et al.*, 1993; Olivetti *et al.*, 1994b, 1996a). These studies confirmed Linzbach's findings and extended the observation from the left ventricle to the right ventricle as well.

Some of studies have demonstrated that adult myocytes can reenter the cell cycle, synthesise DNA and undergo nuclear mitotic division. These phenomena have been documented in animals and in humans, such as in hypoxic rat myocytes (Arefyeva *et al.*, 1985), in the newt cardiac myocytes (Oberpriller *et al.*, 1988; Tate 1989), in ageing rat heart (Anversa *et al.*, 1991; Capasso *et al.*, 1993), in coronary artery narrowing (Reiss *et al.*, 1993; Kajstura *et al.*, 1994), in myocardial infarction (Ebert and Pfitzer, 1977; Capasso *et al.*, 1992a; Joseph *et al.*, 1992; Reiss *et al.*, 1994), in

19

the end-stage cardiac failure of humans (Quaini, *et al.*, 1994) and in the transplanted human hearts (Beltrami *et al.*, 1997a).

Recently, confocal microscope has been used to observe mitotic division of myocyte nuclei on histological sections of paraffin embedded myocardium (Beltrami *et al.*, 1997a). Double stains are performed on the slide with propidium iodide and α–sarcomeric actin antibody. This method allows the unequivocal detection of nuclear mitosis in myocytes. Exclusively, α–sarcomeric actin labels I bands of cardiac and skeletal muscle cells, because it does not cross-react with other actin isoforms (Skalli *et al.*, 1988). The mitotic nuclei of myocytes are centrally located within the cytoplasm. By contrast, interstitial nuclei are isolated and the cytoplasm of interstitial cells is not stained. Based on this difference, it is easy to distinguish the nuclear mitosis of myocytes from that of stromac cells.

Some new fluorescent DNA stains have been used in confocal laser microscope. Among them YOYO–1 iodide is perfect for studying nuclear details and discriminating power between nuclei and cytoplasm in conventional fluorescence microscope (Tekola *et al.*, 1994). At present, no myocyte mitotic determination is reported by this approach in normal and pathological human hearts.

2.5. DNA ploidy patterns of myocytes

As mentioned above, cardiomyocytes can synthesise DNA and undergo mitosis in physiological and pathological situations. However, the results may be differed after these progresses. DNA replication with a block of mitosis forms polyploidization (Ebert and Pfitzer, 1977; Kazantseva and Babaev, 1979; Oberpriller *et al.*, 1983; Shperling *et al.*, 1983; Takamatsu *et al.*, 1983; Arefyeva *et al.*,1985; van der Laarss *et al.*, 1989a; Vliegen *et al.*, 1986, 1990, 1991; Brodsky *et al.*, 1993, 1994; Herget *et al.*, 1997). DNA replication with acytokinetic mitosis leads to multinucleation (Oberpriller *et al.*, 1983; Arefyeva *et al.*,1985; Anversa *et al.*, 1990a; Vliegen *et al.*,

1990, 1991; Brodsky *et al.*, 1991). DNA replication with karyokinesis and cytokinesis results in cellular hyperplasia (Linzbach, 1960; Astorri *et al.*, 1977; Shperling *et al.*, 1983; Arefyeva *et al.*, 1985; Oberpriller *et al.*, 1988; Olivetti *et al.*, 1987, 1988, 1994; Anversa *et al.*, 1990a, 1990b, 1993; Capasso *et al.*, 1993; Grajek *et al.*, 1993; Kajstura *et al.*, 1994; Quaini *et al.*, 1994; Herget *et al.*, 1997). Thus, the issue of nuclear DNA ploidy patterns of myocytes is very interesting, because myocytes belong to the population characterised by different degree of polyploidization and multinucleation.

The observation of nuclear DNA ploidy patterns is depending on the methods. A number of methodologies have been used for the evaluation of DNA content of cardiomyocytes during the last three decades. Autoradiographic analysis of ^{3}H thymidine-labelled tissue has been used to establish whether DNA synthesis in myocytes occurs during embryonic develping (Klug *et al.*, 1995), during postnatal development (Rumyantsev, 1965; Kranz, 1975; Oberpriller *et al.*, 1988; Erokhina, 1992; van Kesteren *et al.*, 1997) and after the imposition of an overload (Grove *et al.*, 1969). This technique offers the possibility to estimate cell proliferation rate, although the questionable reliability of this method has been emphasised (Murat, 1990). Flow cytometric determination has also been used to analyse the changes in DNA content of myocyte nuclei (Takamatsu *et al.*, 1983; Vliegen *et al.*, 1986, 1987, 1990, 1991; Luciani *et al.*, 1991; Joseph, 1992). This technique offers the unique possibility of evaluating whether DNA content in myocyte nuclei is increased and in which phase of the cell cycle the nuclei are. However, a correct determination of a selected cellular population can be obtained neither by autoradiographic approach nor by flow cytometry. Also, it is impossible to distinguish multinucleation from polyploidization by these two methods. Image cytometric determination is a perfect approach that allows the measurement of DNA content on a cell by cell basis, selecting only those belong to the population to be studied (Grabner and Pfitzer, 1974; Ebert and Pfitzer, 1977; Kazantseva and Babaev, 1979; Brodsky *et al.*, 1980, 1985, 1986, 1989, 1991, 1994; Oberpriller *et al.*, 1988; Vasil'eva and Aref'eva, 1988;

21

Rumyantsev *et al.*, 1990; Erokhina *et al.*, 1992; Kellerman *et al.*, 1992; Böcking, 1994; Huhn *et al.*, 1995; Matturri *et al.*, 1995; Kirshenbaum *et al.*, 1996; Herget *et al.*, 1997). The combination of quantitative assessment of nuclear number and DNA content of myocytes permits this approach to evaluate multinucleation and polyploidization of myocytes at the same time. Thus, the nuclear DNA ploidy patterns of myocytes can be obtained exactly.

However, there are two flaws in nuclear DNA ploidy patterns of cardiomyocytes addressed in the literature. Considering the multinucleation, the myocytes with more than two nuclei are less mentioned. Considering the polyploidization, the myocytes locating in subdiploidy and intermediate ploidies are slightly noted. These weaknesses are restricted to understand the alterations of diseased hearts.

2.6. Chromatin bridges

As early as thirty years ago, Nelson-Rees *et al.* (1966) reported the chromatin bridges in a bovine testicular cell line. From then on, the phenomenon of chromatin bridges has been found in animals and in humans. As a rare morphological feature, chromatin bridges can appear in interphase as well as in the mitotic phase.

Several reports have conducted chromatin bridges in congenital dyserytropoietic anaemia (Frisch *et al.*, 1975; Jean *et al.*, 1975, Hiraoka *et al.*, 1983; Prasher and Prasher, 1989; Sansone and Lupi, 1991). The evidences obtained by light and electron microscope confirm the presence of qualitative defects in erythropoiesis in aplastic conditions. Also, chromatin bridges have been found in leukaemic cells. In 1989, Verbunt *et al.* evaluated "buttock cells", leukaemic B cells with a characteristically sharp nuclear cleft seemingly dividing the nucleus into two or more parts. Ultrastructurally, the separate nuclear lobes of buttock cells were connected by chromatin bridges. Takubo *et al.* searched the ring eosinophils in patients with lowered eosinophil peroxidase activity (Takubo *et al.*, 1993). Twelve cases of lowered eosinophil peroxidase activity were found among approximately 600 000

22

blood samples. Ring eosinophils were observed on the peripheral blood smears in 2 out of 12 cases. In both cases, there were some ring-shaped nuclei with a large central nuclear hole and a nuclear ring formed with a thin nuclear chromatin bridges.

Moreover, chromatin bridges can be invoked by some chemical treatments. Triethylenemelamine induced anaphase-telophase chromatin bridges in BHK cells and caffeine could increased the frequency of chromatin bridges (Dulout *et al.*, 1980). Tournamille *et al.* (1982) studied the proliferating human lymphocytes poisoned by methylmercury chloride. They found that the chromosomes, partially decondensed, were covered with protuberances and connected by various chromatin bridges. Platinol (Katoh *et al.*, 1990) and 2,4-diamino-6-hydroxypyrimidine (Chen *et al.*, 1994) can increase in embryonic death. Cytogenetic analysis of first-cleavage metaphases revealed high incidences of chromosomal aberrations including chromatin bridges.

Several experiments were carried out using Chinese hamster ovary (CHO) cells. Dulout and Olivero (1984) observed the effects of adriamycin and mitomycin C on CHO cells. The results showed that chromatin bridges and lagging chromosomes are apparently induced during the S period of the previous interphase. The occurrence of chromatin bridges in anaphase-telophase could be explained by the induction of chromosome stickiness and, to a lesser extent, by the induction of exchange-type aberrations. On the other hand, lagging chromosomes seem to be the result of chromatid or chromosome breaks, because the lagging chromosomes observed were primarily fragments and not whole chromosomes. In 1993, Olivero and Porier published the article "Preferential incorporation of 3'-azido-2',3'-dideoxythymidine into telomeric DNA and Z-DNA-containing regions of CHO cells". Their experiments exploring the induction of chromatin bridges in AZT-treated cells suggest that the analogue may be able to bind to and disrupt the normal functioning of telomeric DNA. Other studies were performed on CHO cells treated with trimethylpsoralen (TMP) + UVA (Rizzoni *et al.*, 1993; Botta and Gustavino, 1997). Chromatin bridges in ana-telophase were induced by an UVA irradiation at 365 nm, which gives rise to both monoadducts and cross-links. These investigations demonstrate that the so-called 'sister chromatid chromatin bridges' (SCCBs) come from a direct effect of photoinduced cross-links in late G2/mitosis.

Additionally, chromatin bridges were also found in atypical stromal giant cells of cervix uteri (Metze and Andrade, 1991), in binucleated hepatocytes (Barni and Scherini, 1991) in a human breast cancer cell line MX-1 (Wolf *et al.*, 1996) and in ulcerative colitis (O'Sullivan *et al.*, 2002). Schmid and Pfitzer (1985) reported briefly this phenomenon in perinatal human hearts. In congenitally malformed hearts double nuclei with chromatin bridges were common in contrast to normal hearts where they were exceptionally rare. Until now, there are no documents concerning chromatin bridges in adult human hearts.

2.7. Aims of the study

By means of image cytometric and confocal microscopic analyses, quantitative evaluations are performed on myocardial cells obtained from adult human hearts both on biopsy and on autopsy. The purposes of present study focus on myocyte nuclear changes in end-stage cardiomyopathies, in order to obtain more details of the following issues: 1) DNA ploidy ranges of myocytes, 2) post-mortem changes in DNA content of myocytes, 3) degree of polyploidization and multinucleation of myocytes, 4) nuclear area of myocardial cells, 5) nuclear DNA ploidy patterns of myocytes, 6) nuclear mitosis of myocytes, 7) myocytes with chromatin bridge and extension. These studies will be useful for understanding the mechanisms of physiological and pathological changes in normal hearts and in idiopathic dilated, ischemic, transplanted cardiomyopathies.

3. MATERIALS and METHODS

3.1. Determination of DNA ploidy ranges

Seventy-four hearts were collected at biopsy from patients who subjected cardiac transplantation for intractable congestive heart failure at the Hospital of Udine from February 1990 to October 1996. Among them, 30 cases suffered from primary ischemic cardiomyopathy, 37 cases with idiopathic dilated cardiomyopathy and 7 cases belonged to other pathologies.

Tissue samples were obtained from the mid section of the lateral wall of left ventricle. The myocardial cells were dissociated by 50% KOH (Grabner and Pfitzer, 1974) and stained with the Feulgen reaction. All the slides were evaluated by a Zeiss microscope using a 40× objective. The images were obtained using a TCM 112-3CCD camera and were digitised on an IBAS image analyser (Kontron, Oberkochen, Germany). The DNA content of 100 fibroblasts and 200 myocytes were measured in each left ventricle.

The ranges of diploidy were calculated by two ways: the mean ± 10% and the mean ± 3SD of IOD of interstitial cells. The values corresponding to 2, 4, 8 and n times of the diploid value were considered as tetraploidy, octaploidy, hexadecaploidy and 2n-ploidy. These values were defined as "ploidy peaks". Contrarily, the values of DNA content located between the ploidy peaks were defined as "intermediate ploidies", i.e. (2c–4c), (4c–8c), (8c–16c) and so on. The differences of DNA ploidy ranges between two calculated methods were compared according to the sum of ploidy peaks (SPP) and the sum of intermediate ploidies (SIP).

3.2. Estimation of post-mortem changes in DNA content

Seven hearts were obtained at biopsy from patients suffered from intractable congestive heart failure. The incidences for cardiac transplantation were idiopathic dilated cardiomyopathy (2 cases), ischemic cardiomyopathy (3 cases) and valvurar cardiopathy (2 cases).

Tissue samples (about 2×1 cm^2) were obtained from the mid section of the lateral wall of the left ventricle. Each specimen was cut into upper and lower parts along to the long axis, and then both of them were divided into eight parts vertical to the long axis. Each blocks contained the tissue from epicardium to endocardium. The first blocks were immediately fixed in 4% buffered formaldehyde. The others were put in 5 ml physiological saline solution in test-tubes. The test-tubes with upper tissue blocks were stored in refrigerator (4°C), otherwise the test-tubes with lower tissue blocks were stored at room temperature (20°C). The specimens were fixed in 4% buffered formaldehyde at 8, 16, 24, 36, 48, 72 and 96 hours after heart explantation, respectively.

Subsequently, routine image cytometric analysis was performed on each specimen, including the isolation of myocardial cells, the Feulgen straining and the determination of DNA content in 100 fibroblast nuclei and 300 myocyte nuclei. Post-mortem changes in DNA content were analysed according to three measures: the integrated optical density, the coefficient of variation in integrated optical density and the sum of intermediate ploidies.

3.3. Patient population

A group of 13 hearts was collected at autopsy within 24 hours after death. The patients (8 males and 5 females) dead not due to primary heart disease or as a cause major risk factors of coronary artery disease, including hypertension, diabetes, obesity, or severe atherosclerosis. In 9 of 13 patients, the death was provoked by a traumatic injury. In the remaining five cases, cerebral haemorrhagia was found in one, pulmonary thromboembolism in two, and sudden death in the last case. In all the patients, the death occurred within five days after hospitalisation. In addition, the autopsy report and the histological examination of all organs excluded diffuse, metastatic malignant neoplasm and chronic inflammatory states. A detailed description of the multiple criteria used to characterise a normal individual and a non pathological heart has been previously described (Olivetti *et al.*, 1991).

Sixty-seven hearts were obtained at biopsy from the patients undergone cardiac transplantation at the Hospital of Udine during the period from February 1990 to July 1996. Among them 37 patients suffered from idiopathic dilated cardiomyopathy with the average duration of heart failure 22 months (ranged from 2 to 65 months). Ejection fraction was 22 ± 8 % (ranged from 10 to 34 %). Coronary arteriography was performed and excluded the presence of coronary artery disease. Other 30 patients were affected by ischemic cardiomyopathy with the average duration of heart failure 15 months (ranged from 1 to 47 months). Ejection fraction was 23 ± 7 % (ranged from 13 to 42 %).

Another group of 23 transplanted hearts was collected at autopsy (Table 1). The mean donor age was 33 years (ranged from 17 to 56 years). Death of the donors was caused by traumatic injury. The mean allograft cold-ischemic time was 178 minutes (ranged from 103 to 267 minutes). The mean age of the recipients at the time of operation was 53 years (ranged from 27 to 68 years). The cardiac indication for the transplantation was: ischemic cardiomyopathy (13 patients), idiopathic dilated cardiomyopathy (eight patients) and hypertrophic cardiomyopathy (one patient). One patient (Case 9 and 22) performed cardiac re-transplantation because of chronic rejection. The mean interval between transplantation and death was 649 days (ranged from 13 to 2558 days). Within six months, the main cause of death was infection (one aspergillosis, two bronchopneumonitis, three myocarditis and one sepsis).

27

Table 1. Clinical data of patients in the transplanted group

Heart number	Cause of transplantation	Recipient age (years)	Donor age (years)	Recipient sex	Donor sex	Survival days	Cause of death
1	ischemic	66	51	M	M	13	bronchopneumonitis
2	dilated	53	29	M	M	20	sepsis
3	ischemic	62	25	M	F	28	bronchopneumonitis
4	dilated	56	17	F	?	28	acute rejection
5	dilated	46	35	M	M	41	myocarditis
6	dilated	27	44	M	M	43	myocarditis
7	hypertrophic	35	25	M	F	46	myocarditis
8	ischemic	62	20	M	F	52	cephalopancreatitis
9	chronic rejection	48	53	M	F	60	acute rejection
10	dilated	50	43	M	F	65	right ventricular failure
11	dilated	59	24	M	M	81	aspergillosis
12	ischemic	60	54	M	M	148	acute rejection
13	ischemic	68	56	M	F	247	chronic rejection
14	ischemic	53	18	M	M	471	chronic rejection
15	ischemic	61	31	M	F	552	malignant melanoma
16	ischemic	59	28	M	M	595	chronic rejection
17	dilated	63	27	M	M	806	acute infarction
18	ischemic	52	21	M	M	1038	chronic rejection
19	ischemic	49	17	M	M	1841	pulmonary adenocarcinoma
20	ischemic	49	36	M	M	1957	chronic rejection
21	ischemic	56	21	M	M	2094	acute infarction
22	dilated	42	30	M	M	2110	chronic rejection
23	ischemic	44	52	F	F	2558	chronic rejection

Three patients died of acute rejection, one patient died of right ventricular failure, and another one died of cephalopancreatitis. After six months, the main cause of death was chronic rejection (seven cases); two patients died of acute myocardial infarction and other two patients died of malignancy.

3.4. Preparation of myocardial cells

Tissue samples were obtained from the mid section of the lateral wall of left and right ventricles. The samples were minced into small fragments of about $1-2$ mm^3 and incubated in 50% KOH solution at 4°C for 24 hours (Grabner and Pfitzer, 1974). Then the KOH solution was decanted. The tissue fragments were rinsed in double distilled water (DDW) at 4°C for one day, during which the DDW was changed 4 times in order to completely eliminate the KOH. 5 ml of cold DDW were added into the test-tubes and then they were vigorously shaken to obtain a good dissociation of the cells. Afterwards, the solutions were filtered through three layers of gauze and were smeared onto slides coated with poly-lysin and air dried. The smears were fixed in 4% buffered formaldehyde for 50 minutes, hydrolysed with 5 N hydrochloric acid for 60 minutes at room temperature and stained with Schiff reagent for 60 minutes.

3.5. Image cytometric measurement

Nuclear number, area, DNA content and DNA ploidy patterns were determined on 103 adult human hearts by means of image cytometric analysis. The stained slides were observed with a Zeiss microscope using a 40× objective. The microscope was connected to an image analyser (IBAS2000, Kontron, Oberkochen, Germany). Only the nuclei corresponding to be well preserved cells were chosen and measured. The segmentation was satisfactory when the nuclear membrane was intact and neither a staining artefact nor an overlap between neighbouring nuclei appeared in the samples. 100 fibroblasts and 200 myocytes were evaluated in each ventricle.

The integrated optical density (IOD) of interstitial cells was calculated and the mean ± 3SD was considered as the reference diploid value (2c). The values corresponding to 2, 4, 8 and n times of the diploid value were considered as tetraploidy, octaploidy, hexadecaploidy and 2n-ploidy. The values of DNA content between these 2n ploidies were defined as intermediate ploidies, i.e. (2c–4c), (4c–8c), (8c–16c) and so on. The sum of intermediate ploidies (SIP) was calculated including subdiploidy (<2c). Mononucleated, binucleated and multinucleated myocytes were recorded one by one. Therefore, nuclear DNA ploidy patterns of myocytes can be available. DNA content of myocytes was evaluated per nucleus and per cell. The total ploidy index (TPI) was used to calculate the total DNA content including intermediate ploidies with the following equation:

$$TPI = \frac{\% < 2c + 2 \times \%2c + 3 \times \%(2c - 4c) + 4 \times \%4c + 5 \times \%(4c - 8c) + 6 \times \%8c}{\% < 2c + \%2c + \%(2c - 4c) + \%4c + \%(4c - 8c) + \%8c}$$

$$\frac{+ 7 \times \%(8c - 16c) + 8 \times \%16c + 9 \times \%(16c - 32c) + 10 \times \%32c}{+ \%(8c - 16c) + \%16c + \%(16c - 32c) + \%32c}$$

$$\frac{+ 11 \times \%(32c - 64c) + 12 \times \%64c + 13 \times \%(64c - 128c) + 14 \times \%128c}{+ \%(32c - 64c) + \%64c + \%(64c - 128c) + \%128c}$$

3.6. Confocal microscopic assessment

Nuclear mitosis, chromatin bridges and extensions were observed on 86 hearts. Among them, 13 cases belonged to normal hearts, 25 idiopathic dilated hearts, 25 ischemic hearts and 23 transplanted hearts. Two paraffin blocks were selected from the lateral wall of the left ventricle and sections were cut at 5 μm thickness. The sections were deparaffinated with xylene (3 min × 2), then rehydrated with 100%

alcohol (2 min × 2), 96% alcohol (2 min), 90% alcohol (2 min) and 70% alcohol (2 min). Then, the sections were rinsed in bidistilled water (1 min) and in running tap water (2 min). Hydrolysis was performed in $2N$ HCl solution for 25 min at 27°C. After being rinsed again with running tap water (2 min) and bidistilled water (1 min), the sections were stained with YOYO–1 iodide solution (1 μl YOYO–1 iodide stock solution, 1.8 ml PBS and 200 μl 0.1N HCl) for 25 min at room temperature (Takola et al., 1996). The stock solution was supplied by Molecular Probes cat # Y-3601. To visualise α–sarcomeric actin, the sections were incubated with a monoclonal antibody to α–sarcomeric actin (DAKO, Denmark) from mouse and post-incubated with tetra-methyl-rhodamine isothiocyanate (TRITC) -labeled anti-mouse IgM.

A DMRB–Fluo microscope (Leica, Germany) was used for standard visual inspection with blue (YOYO–1) and green (α-sarcomeric actin) incident light. Confocal images were obtained with TCS 4D confocal laser scanning instrument (Leica, Germany). A 40× oil objective (numerical aperture of 1.00) was used to observe the mitotic figures, chromatin bridges and extensions. A 100× oil objective (numerical aperture of 1.30) was used to study the detailed chromatin pattern. The total of 10000 myocyte nuclei was observed in each heart. Mitotic figures were observed on YOYO–1 iodide ($\lambda = 488$) stained slides. Myocytes and non-myocytes were distinguished by looking for sarcoplasmic α-sarcomeric actin ($\lambda = 568$). Mitotic images were collected using the line averaging (with eight scans) for noise reduction.

3.7. Statistical analysis

(i) The data were examined by the Shapiro-Wilk's W-test to determine the property of distribution. For normal distribution, the data were presented as mean ± SD, mean ± SEM or mean with 95% confidence interval. For non-normal distribution, the data were presented as median with interquartile range. (ii) The one-way analysis of variance (ANOVA) was used to evaluate the differences among three groups,

31

followed by Tukey test to compare the differences between any two groups. (iii) The paired or unpaired Student's t-test was used to compare the parametric data. (iv) The Wilcoxen matched pairs test and Mann-Whitney U-test were used to compare the non-parametric data between two groups. (v) The chi-square test was used to analyse the occurrence. (vi) The correlation coefficient was used to evaluate the relationship among variables. The p value was considered as significant if less than 0.05. The STATISTICA for Windows (release 4.0A, Statsoft, Inc., 1993) was used to operate all the statistical tests.

4. RESULTS

4.1. DNA ploidy ranges of myocytes

Figure 1 shows six histograms of integrated optical density (IOD) obtained from interstitial cells. Among them, the mean value of IOD was almost same, but the scatter of the diploid peak varied individually, i.e. the standard division (SD) of IOD increased from Case A to F (see Table 2). Thus, the range of the diploid peak of interstitial cells increased as the coefficient of variation of IOD increased from Case A to Case F. A preferable diploid range was calculated according to the mean ± 3SD of IOD of interstitial cells. However, if the diploid range was calculated according to the mean ± 10% of IOD of interstitial cells, some different results were obtained. The diploid range was identical in Case B. The diploid range was enlarged in Case A, or narrowed in Case C to F.

Table 2. Comparison on DNA ploidy ranges between two calculated motheds

Case	IOD mean ± SD	CV (%)	mean ± 3SD SPP (%)	SIP (%)	mean ± 10% SPP (%)	SIP (%)
A	5.000 ± 0.114	2.28	92.5	7.5	96.4	3.6
B	4.996 ± 0.148	2.96	88.7	11.3	88.7	11.3
C	4.998 ± 0.171	3.42	88.3	11.7	87.1	12.9
D	4.976 ± 0.220	4.42	93.8	6.2	86.5	13.5
E	4.998 ± 0.278	5.56	94.0	6.0	80.7	19.3
F	5.000 ± 0.319	6.38	92.8	7.2	69.4	30.6

IOD: integrated optical density of interstitial cells.
SD: standard division of IOD of interstitial cells.
CV: coefficient of variation of IOD of interstitial cells.
SPP: sum of ploidy peaks of myocytes.
SIP: sum of intermediate ploidies of myocytes.

33

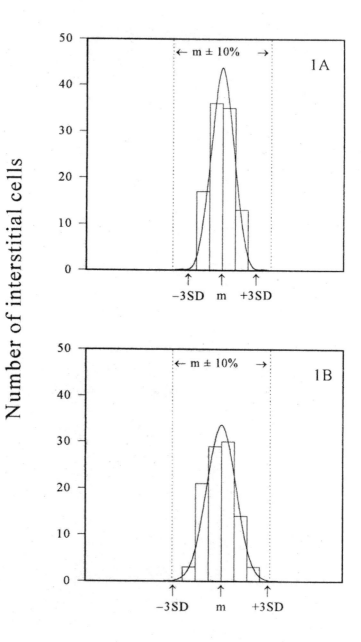

Figure 1A and 1B. Histograms of interstitial cells. Among these 6 histograms, the DNA content shows the same mean value of IOD with different scatter. The CV of IOD increases from A to F. The data are listed in Table 2.

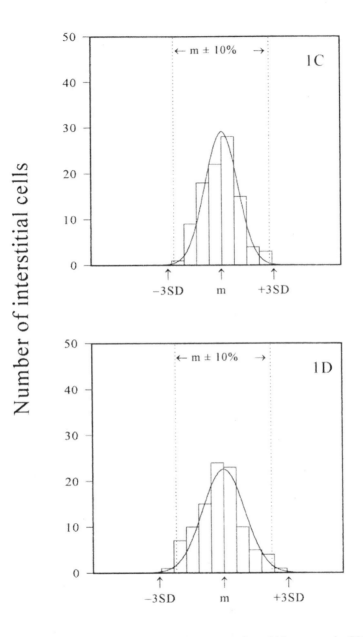

Figure 1C and 1D. Histograms of interstitial cells. Among these 6 histograms, the DNA content shows the same mean value of IOD with different scatter. The CV of IOD increases from A to F. The data are listed in Table 2.

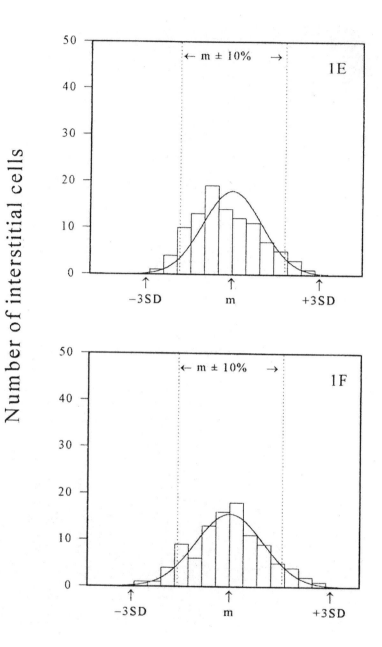

Figure 1E and 1F. Histograms of interstitial cells. Among these 6 histograms, the DNA content shows the same mean value of IOD with different scatter. The CV of IOD increases from A to F. The data are listed in Table 2.

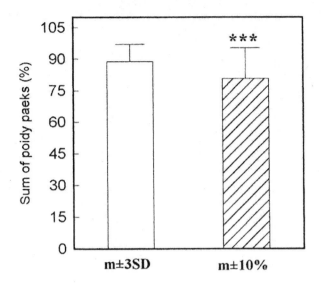

Figure 2. The sum of ploidy peaks (SPP) of myocytes from 74 left ventricles. *** indicates the statistically significant difference at $p < 0.001$ level (Wilcoxon matched pairs test).

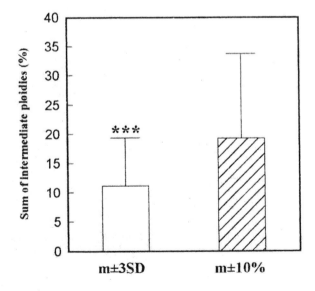

Figure 3. The sum of intermediate ploidies (SIP) of myocytes from 74 left ventricles. *** indicates the statistically significant difference at $p < 0.001$ level (Wilcoxon matched pairs test).

Also, the same phenomena occurred with respect to the ranges of DNA ploidies of myocytes. Table 2 lists the results of DNA content of myocytes from the same cases presented in Figure 1. When the diploid range was calculated according to the mean ± 10% of IOD of interstitial cells, the SPP of myocytes was amplified and the SIP of myocytes was reduced in Case A; whereas, corresponding values of the SPP and the SIP of myocytes changed to the opposite direction from Case C to F. Figures 2 and 3 present the SPPs and the SIPs of myocytes calculated by two methods from 74 cases. On the whole, the SPP of myocytes decreased by 9% and the SIP of myocytes increased by 70% calculated by the mean ± 10% compared to that of calculating it by the mean ± 3SD of IOD of interstitial cells ($p < 0.001$).

4.2. Post-mortem changes in DNA content

Figure 4 shows the integrated optical density (IOD) of nuclear DNA content of interstitial cells at different time intervals after cardiac explantation. When the tissue samples were stored at lower temperature (4°C), the values of the integrated optical density were steady even at 96 hours after cardiac explantation. When the tissue samples were stored at room temperature, the values of the integrated optical density decreased from 48 hours after cardiac explantation. A 7% of decrease in the integrated optical density was found at 72 hours after cardiac explantation ($p > 0.05$). The integrated optical density decreased by 13% at 96 hours after cardiac explantation ($p < 0.05$).

Figure 5 presents the coefficient of variation (CV) of integrated optical density obtained from interstitial cells at different time intervals after cardiac explantation. The coefficients of variation of integrated optical density were fairly stable when the specimens were put at 4°C. Otherwise, when the specimens were put at room temperature, the coefficients of variation of integrated optical density increased as the time extension after cardiac explantation. The coefficients of variation of integrated optical density increased 23% and 47% at 36 and 48 hours after cardiac explantation

($p > 0.05$). The coefficients of variation of integrated optical density increased 1.1-fold and 1.6-fold at 72 and 96 hours after cardiac explantation ($p < 0.05$).

Figure 6 displays the sum of intermediate ploidies (SIP) of myocyte nuclei at different time intervals after cardiac explantation. No significant changes were found in the sum of intermediate ploidies, when tissue samples were kept in refrigerator. However marked increases in the sum of intermediate ploidies were found after 48 hours of cardiac explantation, when tissue samples were kept at room temperature. The values of the sum of intermediate ploidies increased by about 3 times and 5 times at 72 and 96 hours after cardiac explantation ($p < 0.05$).

In summary, no significant changes in nuclear DNA content were found even at 96 hours post-mortem, when tissue samples were stored at lower temperature. If the specimens were kept at room temperature, the alterations of DNA content occur after 48 hours of death. The post-mortem changes in DNA content were characterised by the decrease in the integrated optical density and by the increase in the coefficient of variation of integrated optical density as well as the sum of intermediate ploidies of myocytes.

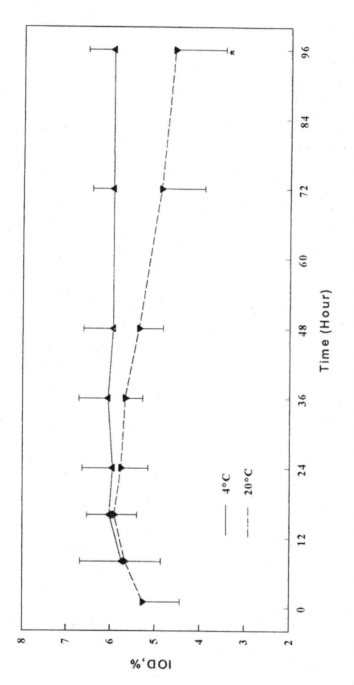

Figure 4. Post-mortem changes in the integrated optical density (IOD) of interstitial cells at different time intervals after cardiac explantation. The data are presented as mean ± SD. The uptriancle with the solid line and the downtriancle with dashed line are the results obtained from the samples stored at 4°C and 20°C, respectively. * indicates statistically different from others, except that of 72 hours at 20°C, at $p < 0.05$ level (paired Student's t-test).

40

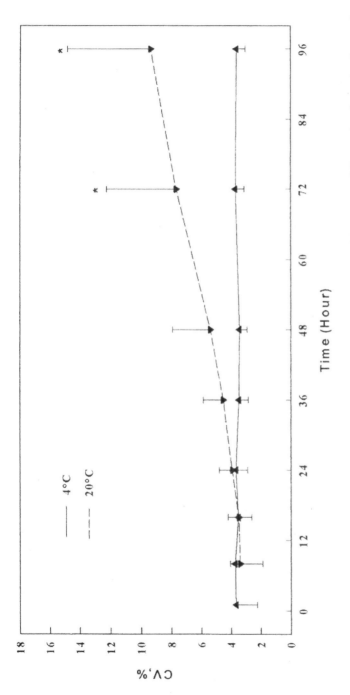

Figure 5. Post-mortem changes in the coefficient of variation of IOD calculated from interstitial cells at different time intervals after cardiac explantation. The data are presented as mean ± SD. The uptriancle with the solid line and the downtriancle with dashed line are the results obtained from the samples stored at 4°C and 20°C, respectively. * indicates statistically different from others at $p < 0.05$ level (Wilcoxon matched pairs test).

41

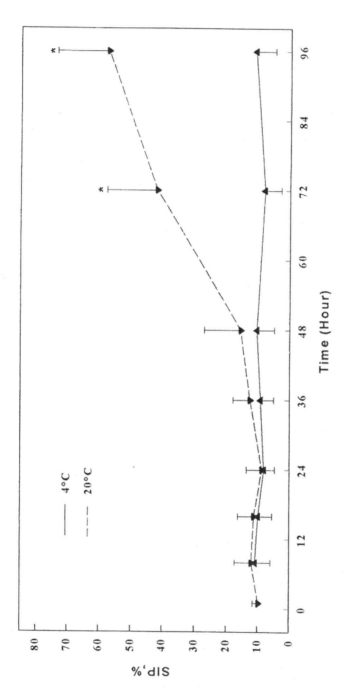

Figure 6. Post-mortem changes in the sum of intermediate ploidies of myocyte nuclei at different time intervals after cardiac explantation. The data are presented as mean ± SD. The uptriancle with the solid line and the downtriancle with dashed line are the results obtained from the samples stored at 4°C and 20°C, respectively. * indicates statistically different from others at $p < 0.05$ level (Wilcoxon matched pairs test).

42

4.3. Anatomical parameters

The gross characteristics in both ventricles are presented in Table 3. Compared to the control group, the heart weight increased by 78%, 83% and 36% in the idiopathic dilated group ($p < 0.001$), ischemic group ($p < 0.001$) and transplanted group ($p < 0.01$), respectively. Furthermore, the left ventricular weight increased about 90% in dilated and ischemic hearts ($p < 0.001$), whereas the increase in the left ventricular weight was less than 20% in transplanted hearts ($p > 0.05$). Augmentation of right ventricular weight was 67%, 82% and 40% in dilated group ($p < 0.001$), ischemic group ($p < 0.001$) and transplanted group ($p < 0.05$), respectively. There was no statistical difference in the thickness of ventricular walls between diseased hearts and control hearts.

4.4. Number of nuclei per myocyte

The percentages of mononucleated, binucleated and multinucleated myocytes in both ventricles are presented in Figure 7. In control hearts, 73.67% of myocytes from the left ventricle were mononucleated, 25.6% of myocytes were binucleated and only 0.73% of myocytes were multinucleated. In the right ventricle, mononucleated, binucleated and multinucleated myocytes were 82.17%, 17.23% and less than 0.6%. It was found only one myocyte with five nuclei.

In the left ventricle of idiopathic dilated cardiomyopathy, the percentage of mononucleated myocytes decreased by 31% ($p < 0.001$) and the number of binucleated, trinucleated and tetranucleated myocytes increased by 57% ($p < 0.001$), 9.7–fold ($p < 0.001$) and 15–fold ($p < 0.001$), respectively. Additionally, rare myocytes had five nuclei (0.15%). In the right ventricle, the myocyte percentage decreased by 26% ($p < 0.001$) in mononucleated population, while binucleated, trinucleated and tetranucleated myocytes increased by 87% ($p < 0.001$), 9.5–fold ($p < 0.001$) and 17–fold ($p < 0.001$), respectively.

In the left ventricle of ischemic hearts, the percentage of mononucleated myocytes decreased by 25% ($p < 0.001$) and the number of binucleated, trinucleated and tetranucleated myocytes increased by 54% ($p < 0.001$), 6.8–fold ($p < 0.001$) and 6.6–fold ($p < 0.001$), respectively. Similar changes occurred in the right ventricle. Numerically, the myocyte percentages decreased by 21% ($p < 0.001$) in mononucleated population, while binucleated, trinucleated and tetranucleated myocytes increased by 77% ($p < 0.001$), 7.4–fold ($p < 0.001$) and 8.2–fold ($p < 0.01$), respectively.

In the left ventricle of transplanted hearts, the percentage of mononucleated myocytes decreased by 16% ($p < 0.01$) and the number of binucleated, trinucleated and tetranucleated myocytes increased by 37% ($p < 0.01$), 3.1–fold ($p < 0.05$) and 2.7–fold ($p < 0.05$), respectively. In the right ventricle, mononucleated myocytes decreased by 14% ($p < 0.001$), while binucleated, trinucleated and tetranucleated myocytes increased by 58% ($p < 0.001$), 2.5–fold ($p > 0.05$) and 1.3–fold ($p > 0.05$), respectively.

In conclusion, end-stage cardiomyopathic hearts were characterised by a decrease in mononucleated myocytes and by an increase in binucleated and multinucleated myocytes in both ventricles. The degree of multinucleation was prominent in dilated hearts and medium in ischemic hearts.

Table 3. Gross Cardiac Characteristics

Characteristic	Control	Dilated	Ischemic	Transplanted
Number	13	37	30	23
Age (years)	42.46±23.21	53.59±10.79	56.64±7.60	54.74±9.67
Heart weight (g)	373.08±72.74	485.89±147.93***	500.29±125.52***	370.78±89.43**
Left ventricular weight (g)	168.62±45.40	315.44±111.90***	314.43±93.92***	198.70±51.95
Right ventricular weight (g)	57.85±21.67	96.50±32.20***	105.54±29.04***	81.17±33.58*
Age (years)	42.46±23.21	53.59±10.79	56.64±7.60	54.74±9.67
Anterior wall	1.59±0.27	1.62±0.45	1.62±0.38	1.78±0.39
Lateral wall	1.58±0.24	1.57±0.49	1.66±0.44	1.74±0.37
Posterior wall	1.53±0.20	1.48±0.40	1.35±0.42	1.67±0.31
Average	1.57±0.20	1.55±0.41	1.54±0.34	1.73±0.33
Thickness of interventricular septum wall (cm)				
Anterior wall	1.56±0.31	1.36±0.39	1.31±0.42	1.57±0.27
Posterior wall	1.58±0.38	1.37±0.39	1.37±0.41	1.57±0.32
Average	1.57±0.33	1.37±0.36	1.34±0.37	1.57±0.28
Thickness of right ventricular wall (cm)				
Anterior wall	0.54±0.24	0.50±0.14	0.60±0.17	0.60±0.15
Lateral wall	0.66±0.23	0.62±0.17	0.71±0.18	0.69±0.19
Posterior wall	0.63±0.16	0.68±0.16	0.69±0.20	0.70±0.20
Average	0.61±0.18	0.60±0.13	0.67±0.14	0.66±0.16

Results are presented as mean ± SD. *, ** and *** indicate statistical difference compared to the control group at the $p < 0.05$, $p < 0.01$ and $p < 0.001$ levels, respectively (unpaired Student's t-test).

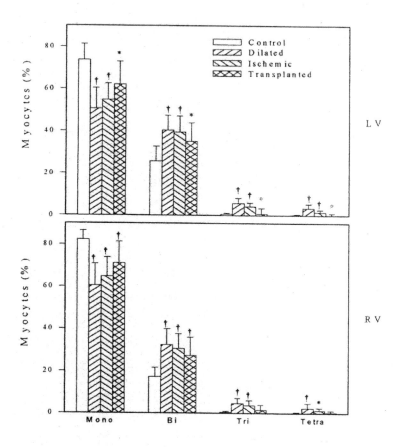

Figure 7. Mononucleated, binucleated, trinucleated and tetranucleated myocytes in left ventricle (LV) and right ventricle (RV). The data are presented as mean ± SD. °, * and † indicate the statistically significant differences from the control group at $p < 0.05$, $p < 0.01$ and $p < 0.001$ levels (Mann-Whitney U-test).

4.5. DNA content of myocytes

4.5.1. DNA content per nucleus

Figure 8 shows the DNA content of myocyte nuclei in the left ventricle. In control hearts, the nuclear DNA content was distributed nearly equally at 2c (43%) and 4c

(47%). The values of intermediate ploidies were very low and the highest ploidy was located at 8c (4.2%).

The most characteristic phenomenon in the dilated group was a significant decrease in the percentage of diploid myocyte nuclei (83%) ($p < 0.001$). Meanwhile, the increase in myocyte nuclei was found in 4c–8c (3-fold, $p < 0.001$) and in 8c (7.8-fold, $p < 0.001$). The distribution of myocyte nuclei shifted towards the higher ploidies, particularly 16c (14%, $p < 0.001$), and, despite a low, but statistically significant number, towards 8c–16c, 16c–32c and 32c ($p < 0.001$). The highest ploidy appeared at 64c.

The nuclear DNA content in the ischemic group decreased from <2c to 4c and increased in the DNA ploidies higher than 4c. The changes were similar to that of dilated hearts, but in a little lower degree. About 8.6% of myocyte nuclei were hexadecaploid ($p < 0.001$) and the highest ploidy appeared at 32c–64c.

In the transplanted group, the most characteristic phenomena were marked increments in the percentages of myocyte nuclei locating in <2c (8.3-fold, $p < 0.001$) and in 2c–4c (3.3-fold, $p < 0.001$). The percentage of diploid myocyte nuclei decreased by 53% ($p < 0.001$) and that of tetraploid nuclei decreased by 20% ($p > 0.05$), whereas 16% of myocyte nuclei had DNA content greater than 4c so that polyploid nuclei augmented two times compared to those of control hearts ($p < 0.01$). The highest ploidy appeared at 16c–32c. Furthermore, the percentage of polyploid myocyte nuclei showed negative relationships with the allograft cold-ischemic time ($p < 0.05$) and with the grade of rejection episode ($p < 0.01$), i.e., when the allograft cold-ischemic time was shorter, or the rejection grade of allograft was lower, the percentage of polyploid myocyte nuclei was higher.

Figure 9 shows the DNA content of myocyte nuclei in the right ventricle. In control hearts, the DNA content of myocyte nuclei was presented as a prominent peak in diploid nuclei (58%) and a second peak in tetraploid nuclei (35%). Only 2% of myocyte nuclei had 8c DNA content.

47

In idiopathic dilated hearts, the change in DNA content of myocyte nuclei was similar to that of the left one, because of a marked decrease of the diploid myocyte nuclei (79%, $p < 0.001$). The myocyte nuclei having DNA content higher than 4c increased significantly, especially in 8c (14-fold augmentation, $p < 0.001$). About 9% of myocyte nuclei had 16c DNA content ($p < 0.001$). The highest ploidy was found at 64c.

In ischemic cardiomyopathy, the diploid myocyte nuclei decreased to 17% ($p < 0.001$). The percentages of myocyte nuclei increased in tetraploidy ($p < 0.001$) and the DNA ploidies higher than 4c, particularly in 8c (12-fold, $p < 0.001$). Hexadecaploid myocyte nuclei were about 5% ($p < 0.001$) and the highest ploidy was found at 32c.

In transplanted hearts, the changes in DNA content of myocyte nuclei in the right ventricle was similar to that of the left one, i.e. marked augmentations of the myocyte nuclei locating in <2c (6-fold, $p < 0.001$) and 2c–4c (2.7-fold, $p < 0.001$), while diploid nuclei decreased by 36% ($p < 0.001$). Moreover, polyploid nuclei (DNA content larger than 4c) increased by 1.5-fold ($p < 0.01$). The highest ploidy was found at 16c.

In conclusion, idiopathic dilated and ischemic cardiomyopathic hearts were characterised by a significant decrease of diploid myocyte nuclei and by an increase in myocytic nuclei with DNA content higher than 4c. These changes were similar in both ventricles and showed a slightly higher degree in dilated hearts compared to those of ischemic hearts. The myopathy after cardiac transplantation was characterised by a significant decrease of diploid myocyte nuclei, by an increase in the myocyte nuclei with DNA content higher than 4c and especially in intermediate ploidies.

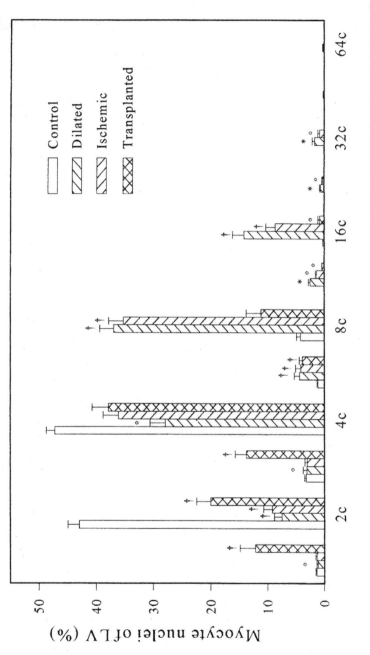

Figure 8. The nuclear DNA content of myocytes in left ventricle. The data are presented as mean ± SEM. °, * and † indicate the statistically significant differences from the control group at $p < 0.05$, $p < 0.01$ and $p < 0.001$ levels (Mann-Whitney U-test).

49

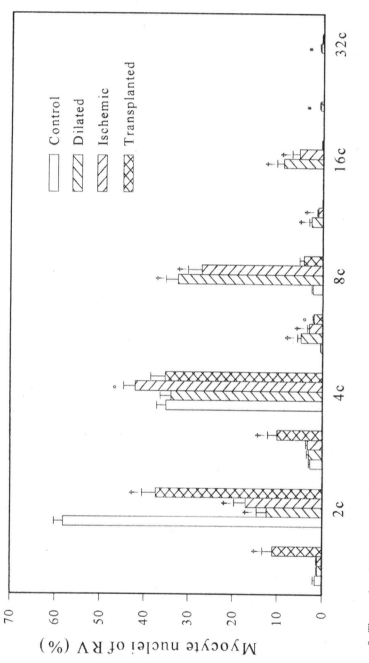

Figure 9. The nuclear DNA content of myocytes in right ventricle. The data are presented as mean ± SEM. °, * and † indicate the statistically significant differences from the control group at $p < 0.05$, $p < 0.01$ and $p < 0.001$ levels (Mann-Whitney U-test).

4.5.2. DNA content per cell

According to nuclear DNA content and number of nuclei per myocyte, we calculated the DNA content per myocyte (the sum of DNA ploidy of every nucleus per cell). Figure 10 shows the cellular DNA content of myocytes in the left ventricle. In control hearts, the DNA content was mainly distributed in 3 peaks: 2c (27%), 4c (50%) and 8c (16%). The highest ploidy appeared at 16c.

In dilated hearts, the percentage of diploid myocytes decreased by 87% ($p <$ 0.001) and that of tetraploid myocytes reduced to 16% ($p < 0.001$). Moreover, an obvious increase was found in 8c (92%, $p < 0.001$) and in 16c (30-fold, $p < 0.001$). The distribution of myocytes went towards higher ploidies, especially in 32c (7.5%, $p < 0.001$). The highest ploidy located at 128c.

Similar changes were found in ischemic cardiomyopathy. The percentage of diploid myocytes decreased by 84% ($p < 0.001$) and that of tetraploid myocytes reduced to 22% ($p < 0.001$). Striking increases were found in 8c (117%, $p < 0.001$), in 8c−16c (7.9-fold, $p < 0.001$) and in 16c (23-fold, $p < 0.001$). Moreover, the distribution of myocytes shifted towards higher ploidies. The highest ploidy located at 64c−128c.

In transplanted hearts, a marked augmentation of myocytes was found in the DNA ploidy class <2c (4-fold, $p < 0.01$) and 2c−4c (3-fold, $p < 0.01$). The percentage of diploid myocytes decreased 58% ($p < 0.001$) and that of tetraploid myocytes decreased by 41% ($p < 0.001$). Meanwhile, the distribution of myocytes shifted towards higher ploidies. A 98% of increase was found in the percentage of myocytes having DNA content higher than 4c ($p < 0.01$). The highest ploidy located at 32c−64c.

Figure 11 shows the cellular DNA content of myocytes in the right ventricle. The distribution of myocyte in the control group was mainly represented by diploid peak (42%) and tetraploid peak (45%). The highest ploidy occurred at 16c. In cardiomyopathic hearts, the changes were similar to those of the left ventricle.

51

In conclusion, both idiopathic dilated and ischemic cardiomyopathic hearts were characterised by an increase in the myocyte having DNA content higher than 4c, biventricularly. These changes were more prominent in idiopathic dilated cardiomyopathy. The myopathy after cardiac transplantation was characterised by a decrease of diploid and tetraploid myocytes, by an increase in the myocytes containing DNA content higher than 4c and by a marked augmentation of the myocytes in subdiploidy and intermediate ploidies.

4.6. Sum of intermediate ploidies

Generally, in control hearts small fractions of myocytes have DNA content in the subdiploidy (<2c) and in intermediate ploidies. We introduced the concept of the sum of intermediate ploidies (SIP) in order to analyse the change in these few values. Figure 12 shows the sums of intermediate ploidies per nucleus or per myocyte in both ventricles. In the control group, the nuclear values of the sum of intermediate ploidies were 5.63 in the left ventricle and 4.68 in the right ventricle, while the comparable values per myocyte were 6.47 and 5.53.

In dilated hearts, the nuclear values of the sum of intermediate ploidies increased by 110% and 158% in the left and right ventricles. Comparatively, the cellular values of the sum of intermediate ploidies increased 1.7-fold and 2.2-fold in the left and right ventricles. All of these differences were highly significant as compared to those of the control group ($p < 0.001$). In ischemic hearts, the changes in the sum of intermediate ploidies were similar to those of the dilated group. However, these modifications revealed less degree in comparison to the dilated hearts.

In transplanted hearts, the nuclear values of the sum of intermediate ploidies increased by 4.6-fold and 3.9-fold in the left and right ventricles. Comparatively, the cellular values of the sum of intermediate ploidies increased 3.9-fold and 3.3-fold in the left and right ventricles. All the differences were statistically significant when comparing with control hearts ($p < 0.0001$).

52

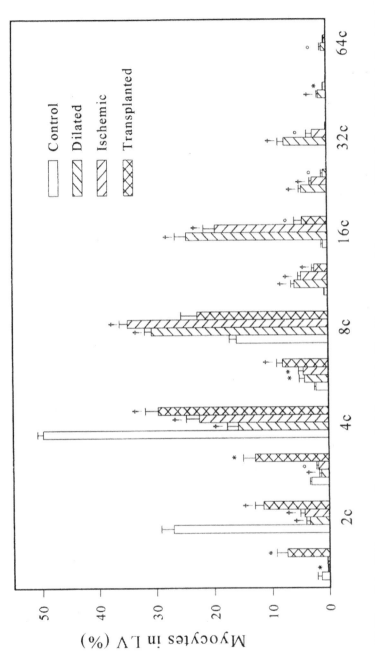

Figure 10. The cellular DNA content of myocytes in left ventricle. The data are presented as mean ± SEM. °, * and † indicate the statistically significant difference from the control group at $p < 0.05$, $p < 0.01$ and $p < 0.001$ levels (Mann–Whitney U-test).

53

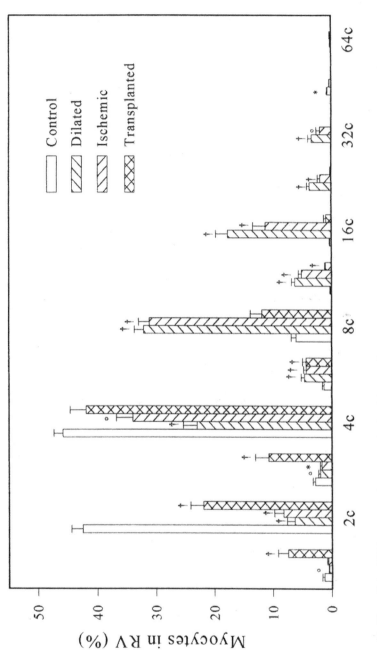

Figure 11. The cellular DNA content of myocytes in the right ventricle. The data are presented as mean ± SEM. °, * and † indicate the statistically significant difference from the control group at $p < 0.05$, $p < 0.01$ and $p < 0.001$ levels (Mann-Whitney U-test).

54

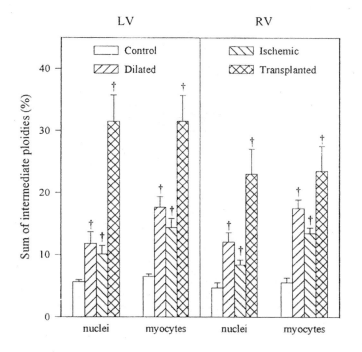

Figure 12. The sum of intermediate ploidies (SIP) in left ventricle (LV) and right ventricle (RV). The data are presented as mean ± SEM. † indicates the statistically significant difference from the control group at $p < 0.001$ level (Mann-Whitney U-test).

Importantly, a strong positive correlation was found between the percentage of myocyte nuclei in subdiploidy and the sum of intermediate ploidies ($p < 0.0001$) in transplanted hearts. The sum of intermediate ploidies became higher as the augmentation of subdiploid nuclei. Also, the sum of intermediate ploidies was markedly correlated with the percentage of apoptotic myocyte nuclei: the larger the number of apoptotic myocyte nuclei was, the higher the sum of intermediate ploidies was ($p < 0.0001$). It was interesting to find out that the sum of intermediate ploidies was correlated negatively to the donor age ($p < 0.01$) and positively to the age difference between the recipient and the donor ($p < 0.02$). The sum of intermediate ploidies increased about one fold, when the donor age was smaller than 30 years ($p <$

0.01) or the age difference between the recipient and the donor was larger than 25 years ($p < 0.05$).

In conclusion, end-stage cardiomyopathic hearts were characterised by an increase in the sum of intermediate ploidies. This feature was most notable in the transplanted group (about 4 times of augmentation).

4.7. Total ploidy index

The total ploidy index calculates the total DNA content including intermediate ploidies. Figure 13 presents the total ploidy index per nucleus and per myocyte in both ventricles. In control hearts, the nuclear values of the total ploidy index were 3.2 in the left ventricle and 2.8 in the right one. The cellular values of the total ploidy index were 3.8 and 3.2 in the left and right ventricles, respectively.

In the left ventricle of the idiopathic dilated group, the values of the total ploidy index increased by 70% per nucleus and by 73% per myocyte. In the right ventricle of dilated hearts, the values of the total ploidy index increased by 75% per nucleus and by 81% per myocyte. In ischemic cardiomyopathy, augmentations of the total ploidy index were 56% per nucleus and 58% per myocyte in the left ventricle. In the right ventricle, corresponding increases in the total ploidy index were 57% per nucleus and 64% per cell. The differences are all significant compared with the control group ($p < 0.001$).

Table 4 shows the results of the linear regression in both ventricles. There were good correlations between heart weight, ventricular weight and the total ploidy index of nuclei and of myocytes: when heart weight or ventricular weight was higher, the values of the total ploidy index were higher. Moreover, when the duration of heart failure was longer, the total ploidy index was higher in the left ventricle ($p < 0.01$), but the same relationship was not found in the right ventricle. No correlations were found between the ejection fraction and the total ploidy index ($p > 0.05$).

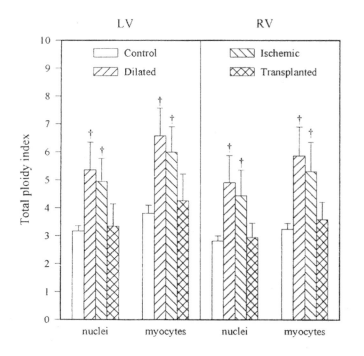

Figure 13. The total ploidy index in left ventricle (LV) and right ventricle (RV). The data are presented as mean ± SEM. † indicates the statistically significant difference from the control group at $p < 0.001$ level (Mann-Whitney U-test).

In the transplanted group, the value of the total ploidy index was 3.4 per nucleus and 4.4 per myocyte in the left ventricle. In the right ventricle, the value of the total ploidy index was 2.9 per nucleus and 3.6 per myocyte. No statistically significant difference was found compared to the control hearts. Moreover, strong negative correlations were found between the percentage of apoptotic myocytes, the sum of intermediate ploidies and the total ploidy index. The larger the percentage of apoptotic myocytes and the sum of intermediate ploidies were, the smaller the value of the total ploidy index was. Also, a positive correlation existed between the donor age and the total ploidy index ($p < 0.01$) and a negative relationship between the age difference between the recipient and the donor ($p < 0.05$). When the donor age was smaller than 30 years or the age difference between the recipient and the donor was higher than 25 years, the value of the total ploidy index decreased about 22%.

In conclusion, the idiopathic dilated and ischemic cardiomyopathic hearts were characterised by an increase in the total ploidy index per nucleus and per myocyte in both ventricles. Compared to control hearts, the total ploidy index increased 60% in ischemic hearts and more than 70% in idiopathic dilated hearts. However, no significant changes in the total ploidy index were found in transplanted hearts.

4.8. Nuclear area of myocardial cells

4.8.1. Average nuclear area

Figure 14 shows the average nuclear area of interstitial cells and myocytes in both ventricles. Considering interstitial cells, the nuclear area of the control group was 84.73 μm^2 and 91.75 μm^2 in the left and right ventricle. In the dilated group, the nuclear area of interstitial cells increased by 35% in the left ventricle ($p < 0.01$) and 29% in the right ventricle ($p < 0.01$) as compared to control hearts. In ischemic cardiomyopathy, the augmentation of nuclear area was 33% and 27% in the left and right ventricle ($p < 0.01$). In the transplanted group, the nuclear area of interstitial cells enlarged of 30% in the left ventricle ($p < 0.01$) and 32% in the right ventricle ($p < 0.01$) compared to control hearts.

Considering myocytes, the average nuclear area of control hearts was 124.88 μm^2 in the left ventricle and 116.43 μm^2 in the right ventricle. In idiopathic dilated cardiomyopathy, a marked augmentation of the average nuclear area of myocytes reached to 1.45–fold in both ventricles. In the ischemic group, the average nuclear area of myocytes increased by 1.3–fold, biventricularly. The differences were statistically highly significant ($p < 0.001$) as compared with control hearts. In the transuplanted group, the average nuclear area of myocytes increased by 39% in the left ventricle ($p < 0.01$) and by 35% in the right one ($p < 0.01$). No significant differences in the average nuclear area of myocytes existed between the left and right ventricles in control hearts or in pathological hearts.

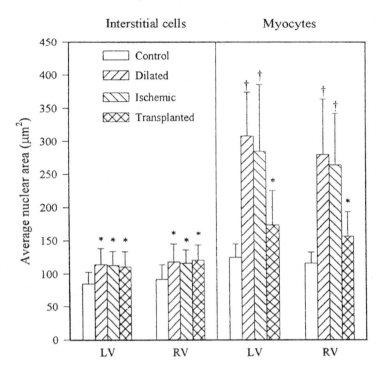

Figure 14 Average nuclear area of interstitial cells and cardiomyocytes in the left ventricle (LV) and right ventricle (RV). The results are presented as mean ± SD. * and † indicate the statistically significant difference from the control group at $p < 0.01$ and $p < 0.001$ levels (unpaired Student's t-test).

Table 4. Results of linear regression

left ventricle	group	equation	number	r value	p value
per nucleus	TPI vs. HW	TPI = 2.71408 + 0.00475HW	70	0.61614	<0.001
	TPI vs. LVW	TPI = 2.97642 + 0.00647LVW	70	0.62146	<0.001
	TPI vs. EF	TPI = 4.56570 + 0.02770EF	63	0.22326	NS
	TPI vs. DHF	TPI = 4.81705 + 0.01905DHF	66	0.31826	<0.01
per myocyte	TPI vs. HW	TPI = 3.58125 + 0.00517HW	70	0.57985	<0.001
	TPI vs. LVW	TPI = 3.92144 + 0.00686LVW	70	0.56966	<0.001
	TPI vs. EF	TPI = 6.25812 + 0.00196EF	63	0.01460	NS
	TPI vs. DHF	TPI = 6.24559 + 0.00283DHF	66	0.32514	<0.01
per nucleus	TPI vs. HW	TPI = 2.67288 + 0.00382HW	70	0.51834	<0.001
	TPI vs. RVW	TPI = 3.58530 + 0.00948RVW	70	0.29511	<0.05
	TPI vs. EF	TPI = 4.21074 + 0.02273EF	63	0.17735	NS
	TPI vs. DHF	TPI = 4.50770 + 0.01007DHF	66	0.16264	NS
per myocyte	TPI vs. HW	TPI = 3.60811 + 0.00361HW	70	0.41925	<0.001
	TPI vs. RVW	TPI = 4.25236 + 0.01131RVW	70	0.30219	<0.05
	TPI vs. EF	TPI = 4.67165 + 0.02125EF	63	0.23873	NS
	TPI vs. DHF	TPI = 5.67228 − 0.00355DHF	66	0.05241	NS

TPI: total ploidy index, HW: heart weight (g), LVW: left ventricular weight (g), RVW: right ventricular weight (g), EF: ejection fraction (%), DHF: duration of heart failure (month).

60

4.8.2. Coefficient of variation in average nuclear area

Figure 15 shows the coefficient of variation in average nuclear area (CVANA), which represents the heterogeneity of the nuclear size.

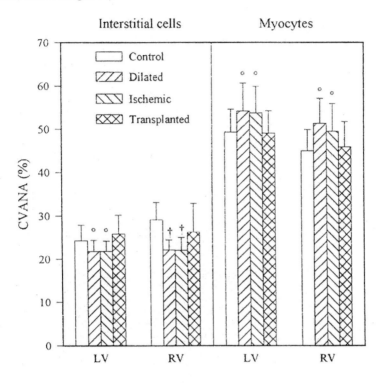

Figure 15 The coefficient of variation in average nuclear area (CVANA) of interstitial cells and cardiomyocytes in the left ventricle (LV) and right ventricle (RV). The results are presented as mean ± SD. ° and † indicate the statistically significant difference from the control group at $p <$ 0.05 and $p < 0.001$ levels (Mann-Whitney U-test).

Considering interstitial cells, the CVANA of control hearts was 24.65% and 29.08% in the left and right ventricle. The CVANAs of interstitial cells were very similar in both ventricles of ischemic and idiopathic dilated cardiomyopathies (about 22%). Therefore, the CVANAs of interstitial cells in cardiomyopathic hearts was reduced by 10% in the left ventricle ($p < 0.05$) and 24% in the right ventricle ($p <$

0.001) compared with those of control hearts. These changes meant that the nuclear size of interstitial cells became homogeneous in dilated and ischemic cardiomyopathic situations. However, no significant changes were found in the CVANA of interstitial cells in transplanted hearts, though this parameter increased by 5% in the left ventricle and decreased about 10% in the right ventricle.

Considering myocytes, the CVANA of control hearts was 49.33% in the left ventricle and 45.01% in the right ventricle. In dilated hearts, the increase in the CVANA was 10% in the left ventricle and 14% in the right ventricle. In ischemic hearts, the CVANA of myocytes increased by 9% in the left ventricle and 10% in the right ventricle. All of these differences showed statistically significant compared to those of the control group ($p < 0.05$). Conversely, no significant changes were found in the CVANA of myocytes in the transplanted group.

4.8.3. Nuclear area of myocytes in different DNA ploidy classes

Figures 16 and 17 show the nuclear areas of myocytes in different DNA ploidy classes of the left and right ventricle, respectively. In the control group, the nuclear areas of myocytes from DNA ploidy classes <2c to 8c were about 70, 90, 110, 148, 190 and 260 μm^2, respectively.

In cardiomyopathic hearts, the alterations of nuclear size of myocytes were revealed in two ways. On the one hand, the nuclear size increased without an increment of DNA content. In each DNA ploidy classes (from <2c to 8c), the nuclear area of myocytes were significant larger (20–62%) than that of control hearts. On the other hand, the nuclear size of myocytes enlarged with the augmentation of nuclear DNA content. Table 5 lists the ratios of the nuclear area of myocytes in different DNA ploidy classes. The ratios of myocyte nuclear area were about 1.3 between the adjacent ploidy classes. The ratios of myocyte nuclear area were about 1.6 between two ploidy peaks. The relative nuclear areas of myocytes can be presented as:

2c : 4c : 8c : 16c : 32c : 64c = 1 : 1.68 : 2.73 : 4.27 : 7.25 : 9.18.

Table 5. Ratios of nuclear area of myocytes in different DNA ploidy classes

Ratio	Control	Dilated	Ischemic	Transplanted
Left ventricle				
2c : <2c	1.27	1.22	1.20	1.22
2c–4c : 2c	1.18	1.27	1.32	1.36
4c : 2c–4c	1.41	1.28	1.24	1.15
4c–8c : 4c	1.28	1.23	1.29	1.32
8c : 4c–8c	1.35	1.35	1.25	1.27
8c–16c : 8c	—	1.20	1.21	1.28
16c : 8c–16c	—	1.40	1.39	1.29
16c–32c : 16c	—	1.15	1.02	1.01
32c : 16c–32c	—	1.29	1.52	—
32c–64c : 32c	—	1.00	1.54	—
64c : 32c–64c	—	0.97	—	—
Right ventricle				
2c : <2c	1.28	1.14	1.27	1.21
2c–4c : 2c	1.30	1.32	1.36	1.37
4c : 2c–4c	1.25	1.24	1.17	1.18
4c–8c : 4c	1.31	1.16	1.29	1.35
8c : 4c–8c	1.38	1.35	1.27	1.31
8c–16c : 8c	—	1.28	1.12	1.22
16c : 8c–16c	—	1.34	1.60	1.15
16c–32c : 16c	—	1.03	0.87	—
32c : 16c–32c	—	1.53	1.67	—
32c–64c : 32c	—	1.43	—	—
64c : 32c–64c	—	1.11	—	—

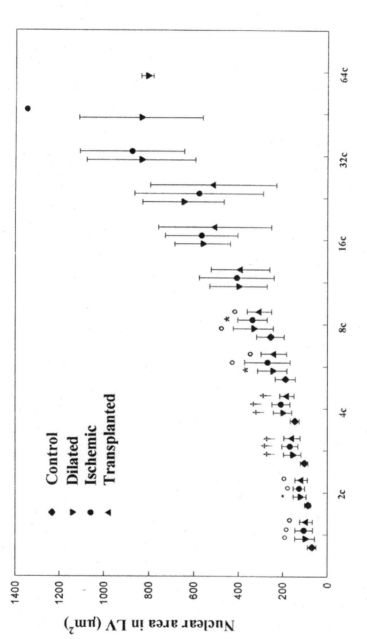

Figure 16. Nuclear area of myocytes in different DNA ploidy classes of the left ventricle. The results are presented as mean with 95% confidence interval . $^{\circ}$, *, and † indicate the statistically significant difference from the control group at $p < 0.05$, $p < 0.01$ and $p < 0.001$ levels, respectively (unpaired Student's t-test).

64

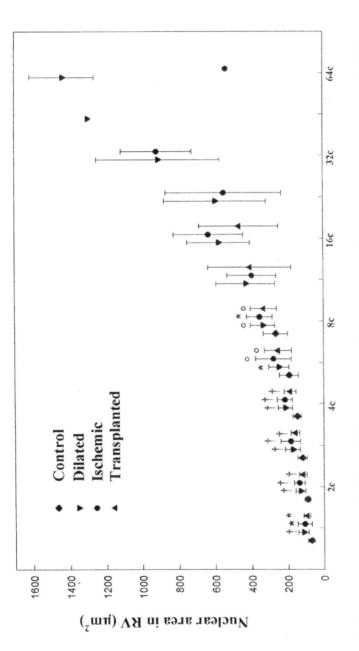

Figure 17. Nuclear area of myocytes in different DNA ploidy classes of the right ventricle. The results are presented as mean with 95% confidence interval. °, * and † indicate the statistically significant difference from the control group at $p < 0.05$, $p < 0.01$ and $p < 0.001$ levels, respectively (unpaired Student's t-test).

4.9. Nuclear mitosis of myocytes

Table 6 lists the results of detecting nuclear mitosis of myocytes. In control hearts, the appearance of myocyte mitosis was rare (in one out of 13 cases), i.e., only one mitosis was found among 130000 myocyte nuclei. In cardiomyopathic circumstances, the occurrence of myocyte mitosis was frequent. In the dilated group, nuclear mitosis of myocytes was detected in 12 from 25 cases ($p < 0.05$), while in ischemic hearts the occurrence of myocyte mitosis was found in 9 out of 25 cases ($p < 0.05$). Numerically, about 15 mitotic figures were found among 250000 myocyte nuclei. Average myocyte mitosis increased by six times.

In cardiac allografts, the incidence of myocyte mitosis increased prominently. Myocyte mitosis appeared in 10 from 12 cases who died within six months after cardiac transplantation. Average mitosis was about 5 among 10000 myocyte nuclei. Comparing to control hearts, augmentation of mitosis was about 64 times in myocyte population ($p < 0.01$). However, the appearance of mitosis decreased sharply (in 4 from 11 cases) after six months of cardiac transplantation. Corresponding average mitosis was 0.8 in 10000 myocytic nuclei. A 9-fold increase in myocyte mitosis was observed in the patients with the surviving time longer than six months after cardiac transplantation, though this difference revealed no statistically significant compared to the control group. Figure 18 shows confocal images of a myocyte undergoing mitosis. Mitotic division in non-myocytic population revealed a behaviur similar to that of the myocytes.

Furthermore, a slight relationship was found between the incidence of myocyte mitosis and the age difference between the recipient and the donor ($p < 0.05$). Numerically, average mitosis of myocytes decreased by 56% when the donor age was smaller than 30 years or the age difference between the recipient and the donor was larger than 25 years ($p > 0.05$).

Table 6. Quantitative analysis of myocyte mitotic division

group	total cases	cases with mitosis	MM among 10000 nuclei
Control	13	1	0.08 ± 0.08
			$0\,(0-0)$
Dilated	25	12†	0.56 ± 0.13
			$0\,(0-1)$
Ischemic	25	9†	0.60 ± 0.23
			$0\,(0-1)$
T1	12	10‡	$5.17 \pm 1.40*$
			$3\,(1-10)*$
T2	11	4	0.82 ± 0.46
			$0\,(0-1)$

T1 group: transplanted hearts with the survival time shorter than 6 months;
T2 group: transplanted hearts with the survival time longer than 6 months
MM: myocyte mitosis. The data are presented as mean $\pm$ SEM and median with interquartile
† and ‡ indicates the statistically significant difference from the control group at $p < 0.05$ and $p <$
0.001 levels (The chi-square test).
* indicates the statistically significant difference from the control group at $p < 0.01$ level (Mann-
Whitney U-test).

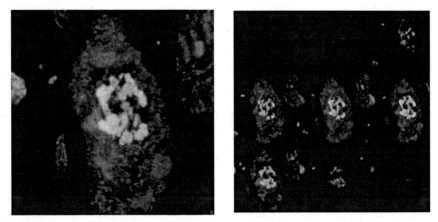

Figure 18 Confocal images of a myocyte mitosis from patient who died 60 days after cardiac
transplantation. The left panel illustrates a larger field area, whereas nine optical sections of the
same cell are shown in right panel.

In conclusion, end-stage cardiomyopathic hearts were characterised by a high

occurrence of myocyte mitotic division. Average nuclear mitosis of myocytes

increased 6-fold in dilated and ischemic cardiomyopathic hearts. Nuclear mitoses of

myocytes appeared prominent in cardiac allografts, especially in the patients who

67

died within six months after cardiac transplantation (a 64-fold increase). By contrast, myocyte mitoses revealed as a declining frequency after six months of cardiac transplantation.

4.10. Variety of nuclear DNA ploidy patterns of cardiomyocytes

4.10.1. Nuclear DNA ploidy patterns of cardiomyocytes

Twelve nuclear DNA ploidy patterns were found in mononucleated myocytes (from subdiploidy to 64c including intermediate ploidies). Table 7 lists 59 nuclear DNA ploidy patterns in binucleated myocytes. 114 nuclear DNA ploidy patterns of trinucleated myocytes were presented in Table 8. 146 nuclear DNA ploidy patterns were found in tetranucleated myocytes (see Table 9). Multinucleated myocytes with 5 nuclei were occasionally seen and 20 nuclear DNA ploidy patterns were found in these myocytes (Table 10).

Table 7. Nuclear DNA ploidy patterns in binucleated myocytes

<2cx2	<2c+2c	<2c+(2c−4c)	<2c+4c	<2c+(4c−8c)	<2c+8c
	2×2c	2c+(2c−4c)	2c+4c	2c+(4c−8c)	2c+8c
		2×(2c−4c)	(2c−4c)+4c	(2c−4c)+(4c−8c)	(2c−4c)+8c
			2×4c	4c+(4c−8c)	4c+8c
				2×(4c−8c)	(4c−8c)+8c
					2×8c

Table 7. Continued in the horizontal way

<2c+(8c−16c)	<2c+16c	<2c+(16c−32c)			
2c+(8c−16c)	2c+16c		2c+32c		2c+64c
(2c−4c)+(8c−16c)	(2c−4c)+16c	(2c−4c)+(16c−32c)			
4c+(8c−16c)	4c+16c		4c+32c		
(4c−8c)+(8c−16c)	(4c−8c)+16c	(4c−8c)+(16c−32c)	(4c−8c)+32c		
8c+(8c−16c)	8c+16c	8c+(16c−32c)	8c+32c		
2×(8c−16c)	(8c−16c)+16c	(8c−16c)+(16c−32c)	(8c−16c)+32c		(8c−16c)+64c
	2×16c	16c+(16c−32c)	16c+32c	16c+(32c−64c)	
		(16c−32c)+(16c−32c)	(16c−32c)+32c	(16c−32c)+(32c−64c)	(16c−32c)+64c
		2×32c...	2×32c	32c+(32c−64c)	32c+64c
					2×64c

68

Table 8. Nuclear DNA ploidy patterns in trinucleated myocytes

<2c×3	2c×3	(2c–4c)×3	4c×3
<2c×2+2c	2c×2+(2c–4c)	(2c–4c)×2+4c	4c×2+(4c–8c)
<2c×2+(2c–4c)	2c×2+4c	(2c–4c)×2+(4c–8c)	4c×2+8c
<2c×2+4c	2c×2+(4c–8c)	(2c–4c)×2+8c	4c×2+(8c–16c)
<2c×2+(4c–8c)	2c×2+8c	(2c–4c)×2+(8c–16c)	4c×2+16c
<2c×2+8c	2c×2+(8c–16c)	(2c–4c)+4c×2	4c+(4c–8c)×2
<2c+2c×2	2c×2+16c	(2c–4c)+4c+(4c–8c)	4c+(4c–8c)+8c
<2c+2c+(2c–4c)	2c+(2c–4c)×2	(2c–4c)+4c+8c	4c+(4c–8c)+(8c–16c)
<2c+2c+4c	2c+(2c–4c)+4c	(2c–4c)+4c+(8c–16c)	4c+8c×2
<2c+2c+(4c–8c)	2c+(2c–4c)+(4c–8c)	(2c–4c)+(4c–8c)×2	4c+8c+(8c–16c)
<2c+2c+(8c–16c)	2c+(2c–4c)+8c	(2c–4c)+(4c–8c)+8c	4c+8c+16c
<2c+(2c–4c)×2	2c+4c×2	(2c–4c)+(4c–8c)+16c	4c+8c+(16c–32c)
<2c+(2c–4c)+4c	2c+4c+(4c–8c)	(2c–4c)+8c×2	4c+8c+32c
<2c+(2c–4c)+(4c–8c)	2c+4c+8c	(2c–4c)+8c+(8c–16c)	4c+(8c–16c)×2
<2c+(2c–4c)+8c	2c+(4c–8c)×2	(2c–4c)+8c+16c	4c+(8c–16c)+16c
<2c+4c×2	2c+(4c–8c)+8c	(2c–4c)+(8c–16c)×2	4c+16c×2
<2c+4c+(4c–8c)	2c+(4c–8c)+(8c–16c)	(2c–4c)+(8c–16c)+16c	4c+(16c–32c)+32c
<2c+4c+8c	2c+8c×2	(2c–4c)+(8c–16c)+(16c–32c)	
<2c+4c+(8c–16c)	2c+8c+16c		
<2c+(4c–8c)×2	2c+(8c–16c)×2		
<2c+(4c–8c)+8c	2c+(8c–16c)+16c		
<2c+8c×2	2c+16c×2		
<2c+(8c–16c)+16c			

Table 8. Continued in the horizontal way

(4c–8c)×3	8c×3	(8c–16c)×3
(4c–8c)×2+8c	8c×2+(8c–16c)	(8c–16c)×2+32c
(4c–8c)×2+(8c–16c)	8c×2+16c	(8c–16c)+16c×2
(4c–8c)×2+16c	8c×2+(16c–32c)	(8c–16c)+16c+(16c–32c)
(4c–8c)+8c×2	8c×2+32c	(8c–16c)+(16c–32c)+32c
(4c–8c)+8c+(8c–16c)	8c+(8c–16c)+16c	
(4c–8c)+8c+16c	8c+16c×2	
(4c–8c)+(8c–16c)×2	8c+16c+(16c–32c)	
(4c–8c)+(8c–16c)+16c	8c+16c+32c	
(4c–8c)+(8c–16c)+(16c–32c)	8c+(16c–32c)+32c	
(4c–8c)+16c×2		
(4c–8c)+(16c–32c)+ 32c		

Table 8. Continued in the horizontal way

16c×3	32c×3
16c×2+(16c–32c)	32c×2+(32c–64c)
16c×2+32c	32c+(32c–64c)×2
16c+32c×2	

69

Table 9. Nuclear DNA ploidy patterns in tetranucleated myocytes

<2c×4	2c×4	(2c−4c)×4	4c×4	(4c−8c)×4
<2c×3+(4c−8c)	2c×3+(2c−4c)	(2c−4c)×3+4c	4c×3+(4c−8c)	(4c−8c)×2+8c×2
<2c×3+(2c−4c)	2c×3+4c	(2c−4c)×2+4c×2	4c×3+8c	(4c−8c)×2+(8c−16c)×2
<2c×2+2c×2	2c×3+8c	(2c−4c)×2+4c+(4c−8c)	4c×3+(8c−16c)	(4c−8c)×2+(8c−16c)+16c
<2c×2+2c+4c	2c×2+(2c−4c)×2	(2c−4c)×2+(4c−8c)×2	4c×2+(4c−8c)×2	(4c−8c)+8c×3
<2c×2+2c+(4c−8c)	2c×2+(2c−4c)+4c	(2c−4c)×2+8c×2	4c×2+(4c−8c)+8c	(4c−8c)+8c×2+(8c−16c)
<2c×2+(2c−4c)×2	2c×2+(2c−4c)+(4c−8c)	(2c−4c)+4c×3	4c×2+(4c−8c)+(8c−16c)	(4c−8c)+8c×2+16c
<2c×2+(2c−4c)+4c	2c×2+(2c−4c)+8c	(2c−4c)+4c×2+(4c−8c)	4c×2+8c×2	(4c−8c)+8c+(8c−16c)+16c
<2c×2+(2c−4c)+(4c−8c)	2c×2+4c×2	(2c−4c)+4c×3	4c×2+8c+(8c−16c)	(4c−8c)+8c+16c×2
<2c×2+4c×2	2c×2+4c+(4c−8c)	(2c−4c)+4c+(4c−8c)×2	4c×2+8c+16c	(4c−8c)+(8c−16c)+16c×2
<2c×2+4c+(4c−8c)	2c×2+4c+8c	(2c−4c)+4c+(4c−8c)+8c	4c×2+(8c−16c)+(16c−32c)	(4c−8c)+16c×3
<2c×2+8c×2	2c×2+(4c−8c)+8c	(2c−4c)+4c+8c×2	4c×2+16c×2	
<2c+2c×3	2c×2+8c×2	(2c−4c)+(4c−8c)×2+8c	4c+(4c−8c)×2+8c	
<2c+2c×2+(2c−4c)	2c×2+8c+(8c−16c)	(2c−4c)+(4c−8c)+8c×2	4c+(4c−8c)+8c×2	
<2c+2c×2+(2c−4c)	2c×2+(8c−16c)×2	(2c−4c)+(4c−8c)+8c+(8c−16c)	4c+(4c−8c)+8c+(8c−16c)	
<2c+2c×2+4c	2c×2+16c×2	(2c−4c)+(4c−8c)×3	4c+8c×3	
<2c+2c+(2c−4c)×2	2c+(2c−4c)×2+4c	(2c−4c)+(4c−8c)×2+16c	4c+8c×2+(8c−16c)	
<2c+2c+(2c−4c)+4c	2c+(2c−4c)×2+8c	(2c−4c)+(4c−8c)+8c×2	4c+8c×2+16c	
<2c+2c+4c+8c	2c+(2c−4c)+4c×2	(2c−4c)+(4c−8c)+8c+16c	4c+8c×2+(16c−32c)	
<2c+2c+(4c−8c)×2	2c+(2c−4c)+4c+(4c−8c)	(2c−4c)+(4c−8c)+(8c−16c)+16c	4c+8c+16c×2	
<2c+2c+(4c−8c)+8c	2c+(2c−4c)+4c+8c	(2c−4c)+8c×3		
<2c+2c+(4c−8c)+16c	2c+(2c−4c)+(4c−8c)×2	(2c−4c)+(8c−16c)+16c×2		
<2c+2c+(8c−16c)+16c	2c+(2c−4c)+(4c−8c)+16c			
<2c+(2c−4c)×2+4c	2c+(2c−4c)+(4c−8c)×2			
<2c+(2c−4c)+4c×2	2c+(2c−4c)+(4c−8c)+16c			
<2c+(2c−4c)+4c+(4c−8c)	2c+(2c−4c)+8c×2			
<2c+(2c−4c)+4c+8c	2c+4c×3			
<2c+(2c−4c)+(4c−8c)×2	2c+4c×2+8c			
<2c+(2c−4c)+(4c−8c)16c	2c+4c+8c×2			
<2c+(2c−4c)+(4c−8c)+16c	2c+4c+(8c−16c)+16c			
<2c+(2c−4c)+8c×2	2c+4c+16c×2			
<2c+4c×3	2c+(4c−8c)+8c+32c			
<2c+4c×2+8c	2c+8c×3			
<2c+4c+8c×2	2c+(8c−16c)+16c+32c			
<2c+(2c−4c)+(4c−8c)+(8c−16c)				
<2c+(2c−4c)+(4c−8c)16c				
<2c+(2c−4c)+(4c−8c)+16c				
<2c+4c×22+(4c−8c)				
<2c+4c+(4c−8c)+8c				
<2c+(4c−8c)+8c×2				
<2c+(4c−8c)+8c+16c				

Table 9. Continued in the horizontal way

8c×4	(8c−16c)×4	16c×4	(16c−32c)+32c×3	32c×4	(32c−64c)×4
8c×3+(8c−16c)	(8c−16c)×3+16c	16c×3+(16c−32c)	(16c−32c)+32c+(32c−64c)+64c		
8c×3+16c	(8c−16c)+16c×2+(16c−32c)	16c×2+32c×2			
8c×2+(8c−16c)×2	(8c−16c)+(16c−32c)+32c×2	16c+32c×3			
8c×2+(8c−16c)+16c					
8c×2+(8c−16c)+(16c−32c)					
8c×2+16c×2					
8c×2+16c+32c					
8c+(8c−16c)+16c×2					
8c+(8c−16c)+(16c−32c)+32c					
8c+16c×3					
8c+(16c−32c)×2+32c					
8c+32c×3					

Table 10. Nuclear DNA ploidy patterns in pentanucleated myocytes

<2c×4+4c	2c×2+(2c−4c)+4c×2
<2c×3+(2c−4c)×2	2c×2+4c×2+(4c−8c)
<2c×2+2c×2+4c	2c×2+4c×2+8c
<2c+2c+(2c−4c)+4c×2	2c+(2c−4c)+4c+(4c−8c)+8c
<2c+2c+(2c−4c)+(4c−8c)+(8c−16c)	4c×2+(4c−8c)×2+8c
<2c+2c+(4c−8c)×2+8c	4c×2+8c×3
<2c+(2c−4c)×2+4c×2	4c×2+8c+16c×2
<2c+(2c−4c)+4c×2+(4c−8c)	(4c−8c)×2+8c×2+16c
<2c+8c×4	(4c−8c)+8c×3+16c
	8c×5

71

4.10.2. Myocytes with nuclei in different DNA ploidies

Figure 19 shows the percentages of myocytes with nuclei in different DNA ploidies. In control hearts, myocytes with nuclei in different DNA ploidies were 1.40% in the left ventricle and 1.47% in the right ventricle. In idiopathic dilated hearts, the percentages of myocytes with nuclei in different DNA ploidies increased by 8.9-fold and 7.8-fold in the left and right ventricles. In ischemic hearts, augmentations of myocytes with nuclei in different DNA ploidies were 6.4-fold in the left ventricle and 5.6-fold in the right ventricle. In transplanted hearts, the increase in myocytes with nuclei in different DNA ploidies was 5.0- fold and 3.8-fold in the left and right ventricles, respectively. All of these differences showed highly statistical significance in comparison with the control group ($p < 0.001$).

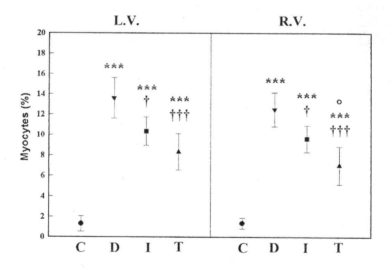

Figure 19: Myocytes with nuclei in different DNA ploidies. The data are presented as mean with 95% confidence interval. The circle: Control group; the down triangle: Dilated group; the square: Ischemic group; the up triangle: Transplanted group. *** indicates the statisticall significant difference in comparison with the control group at $p < 0.001$ level (Mann-Whitney U-test). † and ††† indicate the statisticall significant difference in comparison with the dilated group at $p < 0.05$ and $p < 0.001$ levels (Mann-Whitney U-test). ° indicates the statisticall significant difference in comparison with the ischemic group at $p < 0.05$ level (Mann-Whitney U-test).

4.10.3. Myocytes with nuclei in different intermediate ploidies

Figure 20 displays the percentages of myocytes with nuclei in different intermediate ploidies. In the control group, myocytes with nuclei in different intermediate ploidies were 0.07% and 0.1% in the left and right ventricles. In the left ventricle, the percentages of myocytes with nuclei in different intermediate ploidies increased by 29-, 18- and 11-fold in idiopathic dilated, ischemic and transplanted hearts, respectively. In the right ventricle, the augmentations of myocytes with nuclei in different intermediate ploidies were 12-, 6- and 6-fold in idiopathic dilated, ischemic and transplanted hearts, respectively. All of them presented the statistically significant differences compared to the control hearts ($p < 0.05$).

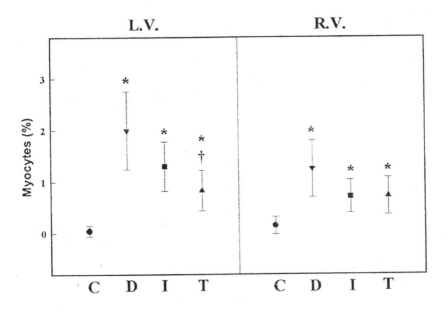

Figure 20: Myocytes with nuclei in different intermediate ploidies. The data are presented as mean with 95% confidence interval. The circle: Control group; the down triangle: Dilated group; the square: Ischemic group; the up triangle: Transplanted group. * indicates the statistically significant difference in comparison with the control group at $p < 0.05$ level (Mann-Whitney U-test).

4.11. Myocytes with chromatin bridge and extension

Our findings confirm that chromatin bridges exist in adult human cardiomyocytes (Panels A-D and G-I in Fig. 21). The slender chromatin bridges may be broken when two nuclei separated or cut during the preparation of tissue section becoming chromatin extensions (Panels E and F in Fig. 21).

Table 11 lists the frequency of cases detected myocytes with chromatin bridge and extension. Among 13 control hearts, myocytes with chromatin bridge were found in 2 cases and myocytes with chromatin extension were found in 1 case. Myocytes with chromatin bridge and/or extension appeared prominent in diseased hearts. Among 25 idiopathic dilated hearts, myocytes with chromatin bridge were found in 17 cases ($p < 0.01$) and myocytes with chromatin extension were found in 16 cases ($p < 0.01$). In 25 ischemic hearts, myocytes with chromatin bridge were found in 14 cases ($p < 0.05$) and myocytes with chromatin extension were found in 7 cases ($p > 0.05$). In 23 transplanted hearts, myocytes with chromatin bridge were found in 13 cases ($p < 0.05$) and myocytes with chromatin extension were found in 16 cases ($p < 0.001$).

Table 11. Detection of myocytes with chromatin bridge and extension

Group	Total cases	Cases with chromatin bridge	Cases with chromatin extension
Control	10	2	1
Dilated	25	17**	16**
Ischemic	25	14*	7
Transplanted	23	13*	16**

* and ** indicate statistical difference compared to the control group at the $p < 0.05$ and $p < 0.01$ levels (the chi-square test).

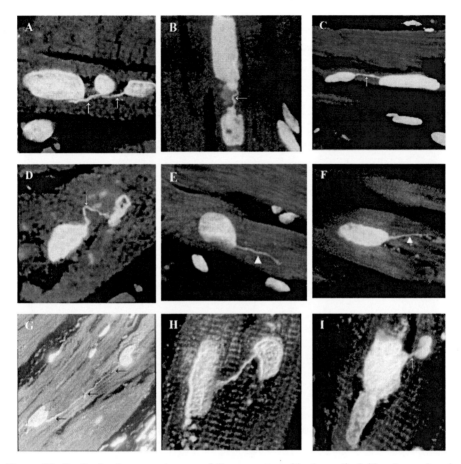

Figure 21: Confocal microscope images of the myocytes with chromatin bridge (arrows) and extensions (arrowhead) from cardiomyopathic hearts. In Panels A-F, green fluorescence shows nuclear DNA stained by YoYo-1 iodide and red fluorescence shows α-sarcomeric actin of myocyte cytoplasm labeled by rhodamine. Panels G-I are 3-dimensional images formed by 9 optical scanning images. (Panels A, B, D, H, I: x100; Panels C, E, F, G: x40).

Figure 22 shows the quantitative results of myocytes with chromatin bridge and extension in the left ventricle. In the control group, myocytes with chromatin bridge and extension were 0.13/10000 and 0.08/10000, respectively. Myocytes with chromatin bridge increased by 24−fold in the dilated group ($p < 0.01$), by 8−fold in the ischemic group ($p < 0.05$) and by 11−fold in the transplanted group ($p < 0.01$), respectively. Correspondingly, myocytes with chromatin extension increased by

75

35–fold in the dilated group ($p < 0.01$), by 6–fold in the ischemic group ($p > 0.05$) and by 13–fold in the transplanted group ($p < 0.01$), respectively.

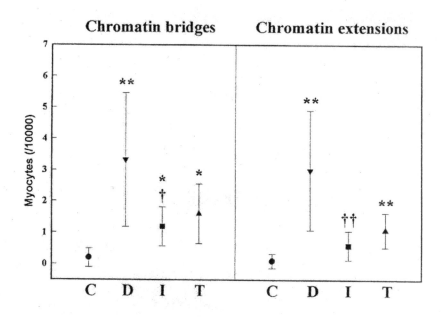

Figure 22: Myocytes with chromatin bridge and extension. The data are presented as mean with 95% confidence interval. The circle: Control group; the down triangle: Dilated group; the square: Ischemic group; the up triangle: Transplanted group. * and ** indicate the statistical significance in comparison with the control group at $p < 0.05$ and $p < 0.01$ levels (Mann-Whitney U-test). † and †† indicate the statistical significance in comparison with the dilated group at $p < 0.05$ and $p < 0.01$ levels (Mann-Whitney U-test).

5. DISCUSSION

5.1. DNA ploidy ranges of cardiomyocytes

DNA ploidy analysis has been applied in the studies on myocardial cells in animals (Bogenrann and Eppenberger, 1980; Brodsky *et al.*, 1980, 1985, 1986, 1988, 1990; van der Laarse 1987; Vliegen *et al.*, 1990; Panizo-Santos *et al.*, 1995) and in humans (Ebert and Pfitzer, 1977; Takamatsu *et al.*, 1983; Adler, 1986; Hayashi *et al.*, 1986; Vliegen *et al.*, 1986, 1990, 1991; van der Laase *et al.*, 1989a; Rumyantsev *et al.*, 1990; Luciani *et al.*, 1991; Brodskii *et al.*, 1989, Brodsky *et al.*, 1993, 1994; Matturri *et al.*, 1995). As DNA content is assessed according to the integrated optical density (IOD) by either flow or image cytometry, reference standard cells are necessary (Munck-Wikland *et al.*, 1990; Coen *et al.*, 1992). It is widely accepted that interstitial cells serve as the internal diploid cells when evaluating DNA content of myocytes. In general, the range of diploid cells is defined from 0.9 to 1.1 of DNA index (DI) (Marchevsky *et al.*, 1996). This range statistically corresponds to the mean $\pm$ 10% of integrated optical density (IOD) of the diploid reference cells.

Theoretically, all non-cycling cells should have the same value on the DNA content (absorbency or fluorescence) scale. Inevitable minimal variations will occur due to slight variations in preparation, staining, and measurement techniques, leading to some scatter around a mean (Carey, 1994). This scatter can be quantified as a coefficient of variation (CV), i.e. the standard deviation divided by the mean value. As presented herein, the CV significantly affects the accuracy of DNA ploidy ranges of myocytes. The different dispersion of diploid peak is ignored, if the mean $\pm$ 10% of IOD of interstitial cells is used as the diploid range. In fact, the CV of IOD may be different from one to another, although the mean value of IOD is the same. Therefore, it is better to consider both the mean and the CV of IOD together when calculating the DNA ploidy ranges in myocardial cells.

It is important to carefully define the DNA ploidy ranges, because myocytes are polyploid population. If not, myocyte nuclei will be classified into either ploidy peaks or intermediate ploidies. As a result, the sum of intermediate ploidies (SIP) will increase and the sum of ploidy peaks (SPP) will decrease, or vice verse. According to Chebyshev's theorem and the empirical rule, 99.7% variations will be encompassed within three standard deviations (3SD) of the mean (Johnson, 1992). Also, in the usual way from the complete available sample, limits are typically set at mean ± 3SD. Values outside these limits are considered as outliers (Healy, 1979) and belong to other class. Thus, using the mean ± 3SD of IOD as the diploid range can preferably define DNA ploidy classes of myocytes. In this way, we have successfully analysed the alterations of DNA content of myocytes in end-stage dilated and ischemic cardiomyopathies of human hearts (Beltrami et al., 1997b).

A number of factors can influence the reactivity of the Feulgen stain in image cytometry (Reith et al., 1994). Generally speaking, the older the material is, the larger the problem of getting well preserved nuclei is. A major problem comes from the fixation. If tissue samples are fixated under low pH conditions for a long time, the destruction of chromatin/DNA will occur. Therefore, the stained nuclei become faint and the CV of IOD increases. In this condition, the sum of intermediate ploidies of myocytes will significantly increase, when using the mean ± 10% of IOD as the diploid range. However, the use of the mean ± 3SD of IOD as the diploid range can overcome this defect so that old materials can be measured (Beltrami et al., 1997b, Yan et al., 1998, 1999b).

In summary, the coefficient of variation influences significantly the range of DNA ploidy distribution. Thus, not only the mean but also the coefficient of variation of IOD would be considered when calculating the DNA ploidy ranges. Using the mean ± 3SD of IOD of interstitial cells as the diploid range can preferably define the ranges

78

of DNA ploidy classes of myocytes. By this way, DNA content of myocardial cells can be estimated in different pathological conditions. Also, it is possible to use old tissue samples.

5.2. Post-mortem changes in DNA content

The performance of cardiac transplantation provides the possibility of systematic studies on post-mortem changes in DNA content of myocytes using bioptic human hearts. In the present study, the post-mortem changes in DNA content of myocardial cells are estimated at different temperature and time intervals. The changes in DNA content are clearly represented by three measures, i.e. the integrated optical density, the coefficient of variation in the integrated optical density and the sum of intermediate ploidies.

The temperature is a sensitive condition on post-mortem changes in DNA content. The results herein demonstrate that the alterations of DNA content of myocardial cells are affected by the temperature of storage for tissue samples. If the specimens are kept at lower temperature (4°C), no changes are found in the integrated optical density (IOD), the coefficient of variation (CV) in IOD and the sum of intermediate ploidies (SIP) even on the fourth day after death. Comparatively, the changes in DNA content occur when tissue samples are stored at room temperature. Within two days post-mortem, limited alterations are found in the IOD, the CV of IOD and the SIP. However, these changes become apparent after two days of death. The IOD decreases, whereas the CV of IOD and the SIP increase. All of them indicate significant reduction of nuclear DNA content.

In view of different variables for detecting the post-mortem changes in DNA content, the CV of IOD is more sensitive than others. After 24 hours of death, this variable increases firmly as the extension of post-mortem time. Otherwise, the changes in the IOD and the SIP appear marked after 48 hours of death.

In summary, the post-mortem changes in DNA content of myocardial cells are characterised by the decrease in the integrated optical density, by the increase in the coefficient of variation of integrated optical density and in the sum of intermediate ploidies of myocytes. No significant changes in DNA content of myocardial cells are found within 48 hours after death.

5.3. Multinucleation and cardiomyopathies

There are some reports that adult ventricular myocytes in the human myocardium are mostly characterised by a single nucleus (Hort, 1953; Adler and Sandritter, 1971; Korecky *et al.* 1979). However, the present study demonstrates that one fourth of myocytes are multinucleated in the left ventricle of control hearts; in the right ventricle 18% of myocytes are multinucleated. Among the multinucleated myocyte population, most myocytes have two nuclei and only small fraction of myocytes have more than two nuclei.

The degree of multinucleation of cardiomyocytes is differant in the literature. A high frequency of binucleated myocytes has been reported by Brodsky *et al.* (1991). In the left ventricle of normal hearts, the mean percentage of binucleated myocytes is 61 ± 3%, 63 ± 4% and 54 ± 5% in the external, middle and inner layer of the anterior wall. By contrast, Olivetti *et al.* (1996b) show that mononucleated, binucleated, trinucleated and tetranucleated myocytes comprise 74%, 25.5%, 0.4% and 0.1% of the entire myocyte population in the control left ventricle. Aging, myocardial hypertrophy and ischemic cardiomyopathy do not affect the proportion of mononucleated and multinucleated myocyte in the ventricular myocardium.

The current numerical analyses of nuclear number per myocyte demonstrate that the degree of multinucleation of myocytes in control hearts is similar to that reported by Olivetti and co-workers (1996b). But the binucleated and multinucleated myocytes increase in the cardiomyopathic circumstances, as agreed with previous studies (Hort,

1953; Adler and Sandritter, 1971; Baroldi et al., 1967; Adler, 1986; Vliegen et al., 1990, 1991; Adler, 1991; Grajek et al., 1993; Kawaguchi et al., 2008). These observations suggest that end-stage cardiomyopathies are coupled with a high degree of myocytic multinucleation, which is considered as a function of increase in cell size. Animal experiments indicate that, associated with the multinucleation, there is an increase in the DNA, RNA and protein content as well as in the ratios of RNA to DNA and protein to RNA (Reasor et al., 1982).

In diseased hearts, it is clear that a decrease in mononucleated myocytes is coupled with an increase in multinucleated myocytes (Beltrami et al., 1997b, Yan et al., 1998, 1999b). The reasons for this phenomenon may be explained considering three different mechanisms: (i) the death of mononucleated myocytes might result in a relative increase in multinucleated myocytes; (ii) the multinucleated myocytes may be formed by the fusion of mononucleated myocytes, which phenomenon has been described during senescence (Anversa et al., 1991); (iii) the increase in multinucleated myocytes resulted from nuclear mitosis without cytoplasmic division.

Until now there are no documents demonstrating that mononucleated myocytes are more sensitive to injurious factors in pathological states, which may lead up to a relative increase in multinucleated myocytes. In addition, we can not exclude that the fusion of mononucleated myocytes may occur during these pathological circumstances. Importantly, evidences have been accumulated that adult ventricular myocytes can be stimulated to synthesise DNA (Linzbach, 1960; Astorri et al., 1971; Rumyantsev and Kassem, 1976; Claycomb and Moses, 1985, 1988; Marino et al., 1991; Capasso et al., 1992a; Grajek et al., 1993; Quaini et al., 1994; Di Loreto et al., 1995; Beltrami et al., 1997a) and nuclear mitosis has been observed in cardiomyocytes (Kazantseva and Babaev, 1977; Anversa et al., 1991; Reiss et al., 1993; Quaini et al., 1994; Beltrami et al., 1997a ; Kajstura et al., 1998). Also, the present study reveals that the occurrence and the frequency of myocyte mitosis are significant higher in diseased hearts. Some studies support that multinucleation in myocytes is mainly due to acytokinetic mitosis, i.e. nuclear poly-mitotic division without cytoplasmic division, which results in the absolute increase in multinucleated myocytes (Brodsky et al., 1980; Petrashchuk and Oniskchenko, 1987).

In summary, end-stage cardiomyopathic hearts are characterised by a decrease in mononucleated myocytes and by an increase in binucleated as well as multinucleated myocytes. The degree of multinucleation is prominent in idiopathic dilated hearts, middle in ischemic hearts and limit in transplanted hearts.

5.4. Polyploidization and cardiomyopathies

Cytokinesis is the last step of cell division that physically separates the daughter cells. Thus, it ensures the proper inheritance of both nuclear and cytoplasmic contents. Polyploidy is essential for cellular differentiation and function in some contexts, however, polyploidy can result from cytokinesis failure and may contribute to the development of pathologies. Consequently, the degree of ploidy and the achievement of cytokinesis must be tightly regulated throughout an organism and among different cell types (Lacroix and Maddox, 2012).

The phenomenon of polyploidization is well known in the field of cardiac physio-pathology, both experimentally in animals and in humans (Sandritter and Scomazzoni, 1964; Adler and Sandritter, 1971; Ebert and Pfitzer, 1977; Kazantseva and Babaev, 1979; Brodsky et al., 1980, 1991, 1994; Shperling et al., 1983; Rumyantsev et al., 1990; Luciani et al., 1991; Vliegen et al., 1991; Kawaguchi et al., 2008). Polyploidization of cardiomyocytes is an essential component of heart growth in the warm-blooded vertebrates with a wide variety (Martynova et al., 2002). The present results obtained from control adult hearts are similar to those published by Takamatsu et al. (1983), although there are some differences existing in the fractions of diploid and tetraploid nuclei in the left ventricle.

There is no doubt that a high degree of nuclear polyploidization exists in cardiomyopathic hearts. In the left ventricle, the percentage of polyploid myocyte nuclei (with DNA content higher than 4c) increases by 10.4-fold, 8.5-fold and 2.1-fold in dilated, ischemic and transplanted hearts compared with control hearts, respectively. In the right ventricle, corresponding value enlarges 18.8-fold, 13.5-fold and 1.5-fold in dilated, ischemic and transplanted hearts, respectively (Beltrami et al., 1997b, Yan et al., 1998, 1999b).

Brodsky and co-workers emphasised that ploidy is a characteristic of the cell and the analysis of ploidy of cardiac myocytes and other cells cannot be made without considering the number of nuclei in cells (Brodsky et al., 1991). A diploid binucleated cell does not differ in its functional characteristics from a mononucleated tetraploid cell of the same type (Brodsky et al., 1985). Accordingly, we estimate the myocyte DNA content, i.e. the sum of ploidies of each nucleus. Thus, the degree of cellular polyploidization is enhanced by the increased level of multinucleation. Considering different pathological situations, the increase in cellular polyploidization reveals high level in the idiopathic dilated group, middle level in the ischemic group and low level in the transplanted group. In the left ventricle, the percentage of polyploid myocytes (with DNA content higher than 4c) increases by 3.1-fold, 2.7-fold and 98% in dilated, ischemic and transplanted hearts compared with control hearts, respectively. In the right ventricle, corresponding value enlarges 7.9-fold, 6.2-fold and 1.3-fold in dilated, ischemic and transplanted hearts, respectively. These results are consistent with other finding that DNA ploidy level (> 8c) as well as the proportion of aneuploid myocyte nuclei were increased in infarcted hearts (Herget et al., 1977).

In the present work we evaluate the changes in DNA content of myocytes in the end-stage cardiomyopathies (Beltrami et al., 1997b). Adler has investigated the changes in the myocardium of hypertrophied human hearts without or with insufficiency: the heart muscle nuclei show a polyploidization which is correlated with myocardial weight. In insufficient hearts of patients suffering from myocardial hypertrophy, the increase in the total DNA content is significantly lower as compared to non-insufficient hearts. The mean ploidy level increases in the cases with lower weights of the myocardium and decrease in the bigger weights in comparison with non-insufficient hearts of the same weights. In contrast to this, the increase in the heart muscle cells is significantly reduced. A lack of contractile proteins, decreased DNA synthesis, increased sclerosis and, in particular, the reduced number of cardiac muscle cells are considered as essential factors for cardiac insufficiency (Adler 1986).

Some observations indicate that in human infarcts, entrance of cardiomyocytes into the cell cycle is transient and that endomitosis, leading to polyploidy, rather than mitosis, leading to karyokinesis, is the final fate of cycling cells (Meckert *et al.*, 2005). The polyploidization in the heart could be genetically programmed (Brodsky *et al.*, 1986, 1988). The growth of the myocytes outside the cycle is, predominantly, function-dependent. Polyploidy is a physiological event in normal heart and it is probably related to the myoglobin and/or protein content of the myocytes. In this way, polyploidy, hypertrophy and cardiac growth are different steps of the same phenomenon. In fact, polyploid cells are capable of highly functional activities within a short period of time, because of the positive correlation between the DNA mass and the cytoplasmic mass (Nagl, 1990). Polyploid myocytes can result from interruption of mitosis (or block of spindle function), which is the most frequent mechanism of polyploidization in mammalian cells. This mechanism of active DNA replication leading to true polyploidization may explain the extremely elevated activity of PCNA observed in the myocytes in the end-stage cardiomyopathies (Quaini *et al.*, 1994; Reiss *et al.*, 1994) and in transplanted hearts (Beltrami *et al.*, 1997a). Compensatory cardiomyocyte polyploidy is a periodical phenomenon in transplanted hearts (Nozyński et al., 2009).

The degree of nuclear or cellular polyploidization of myocytes is correlated with the heart weight and the ventricular weight. Comparising of the DNA content (Feulgen reaction) and total protein content (naphtol yellow S staining) in the same cardiac myocyte, DNA ploidy and protein content grow in a correlated way. The averrage values of cellular area and protein content for tetraploid cells are 1.5 times higher than that for diploid ones (Erokhina *et al.*, 1995). The weight of the muscle tissue may be increased from 30% to twice, depending on the myocyte ploidy of a given myocardium (Brodsky *et al.* 1993). Thus, polyploidization of cardiac myocytes and their post-mitotic growth enhance the heart weight in normal circumstances and create a growth reserve for hypertrophy under pathological conditions.

It would be mentioned that the present estimations are performed on the specimens obtained from the leteral wall including endocardium and epicardium. The nuclear DNA content of myocytes in different sites of the left free ventricular wall has been studied in five hearts affected by dilated cardiomyopathy. All of the different sites reveal diploid and tetraploid DNA content. Variable is the presence of octaploid peak: specifically 40% in the external third, 47% in the medium third and 73% in the inner third. Hexadecaploid peak are revealed only twice and exactly in one medium third and in one inner third. These data, even if quite preliminary, suggest the presence of an increasing gradient of polyploidisation from the external toward the inner part of the left ventricular wall (Luciani *et al.*, 1991). On contrastly, the mean myocyte ploidy in different layers of the anterior wall is similar: in the external layer it is 5.1 ± 0.3 c, in the middle layer 5.5 ± 0.3 c and in the inner layer 4.8 ± 0.4 c. Myocyte ploidy in tissue from the posterior wall of the left ventricle also varies, but is always higher than that of the same layer of the anterior wall (Brodsky *et al.*, 1991).

In summary, end-stage cardiomyopathic hearts are characterised by an increased degree of polyploidization. This feature indicates evident in idiopathic dilated and ischemic hearts and limit in tranplanted hearts.

5.5. Intermediate ploidies and cardiomyopathies

The intermediate ploidies may result from three aspects: (i) DNA synthesis, (ii) DNA lysis and (iii) abnormal mitosis. For example, a myocyte has two nuclei locating in 2c and 4c, respectively. The nuclei might go into ploidy classes (2c–4c) and (4c–8c) by means of DNA replication or retreat into ploidy classes <2c and (2c–4c) by means of DNA lysis. The third aspect will be discussed latterly. Thus, the interpretation of intermediate ploidies seems complicated, because the nuclear growth interweaves with the nuclear damage.

In the idiopathic dilated and ischemic groups, the increases in intermediate ploidies of myocyte nuclei are accompanied by a decrease in subdiploidy (<2c). In this condition, the increase in intermediate ploidies results mainly from the DNA synthesis, i.e., they represent the nuclei in S phase (Beltrami *et al.*, 1997b). This argument is supported by other results, such as the decrease in diploid nuclei, the increase in polyploid nuclei, the high values of total ploidy index and so on. Considering myocytes, the increase in the sum of intermediate ploidies was more marked in pathological situations, particularly in dilated hearts. These aspects result mainly from the high degree of multinucleation and the heterogeneity of nuclear DNA ploidies among multinucleated myocytes, i.e., intermediate ploidies. However, over the past decade, a genetic basis has been partially uncovered in both inherited and hitherto idiopathic dilated cardiomyopathies (Lakdawala *et al.*, 2012), where mutations have been found in genes encoding cystoskeletal, sarcomeric, nuclear membrane, and sarcoplasmic reticulum proteins (Olson, 2006; Brouwer *et al.*, 2011). Therefore, the increase in intermediate ploidies may partially represent the abnormal DNA content.

On the contrary, the sum of intermediate ploidies in transplanted hearts shows strong correlation with the percentage of subdiploidy ($p < 0.0001$), so the marked augmentation of intermediate ploidies indicates the cell injury and DNA fragmentation (apoptosis). As the sum of intermediate ploidies shows close

86

relationship in both ventricles ($p = 0.0015$), we conclude that the degree of myocyte injury is similar biventricularly (Yan *et al.*, 1998, 1999b).

The structure-function correlations confirm that the transition of compensated hypertrophy to heart failure occurs by fibrosis and myocyte degeneration (Hein *et al.*, 2003). Cardiac myocyte apoptosis and necrosis are prominent features of the major cardiac syndromes. Accordingly, the recognition of necrosis as a regulated process mandates a reexamination of cell death in the heart. Over the past decade, however, experiments in Caenorhabditis elegans and mammalian cells have revealed that a significant proportion of necrotic death is, in fact, actively mediated by the doomed cell (Kung *et al.*, 2011). Programmed cell elimination is an important pathological mediator of disease. Multiple pathways to programmed cell death have been delineated, including apoptosis, autophagy and programmed necrosis (Kostin, 2005; Dorn, 2010).

Both necrosis and apoptosis induced by cytotoxic-mediated rejection contribute to the loss of DNA. Therefore, the distribution of myocytes shifts towards lower DNA ploidy classes. The present results obtained by image cytometry agree with previous studies using flow cytometry (Darzynkiewicz *et al.*, 1992), by means of which the fragmentation of DNA (apoptosis) can be detected as subdiploid peak. However, myocytes are polyploid population. The DNA content of myocytes decreases and the distribution of myocytes shifts to the previous lower ploidy when myocytes are injured. For example, damaged diploid myocytes appear in the subdiploid peak, damaged tetraploid myocytes locate in 2c–4c, and so on. According to the current results, the percentages of myocyte nuclei are about equal in <2c and 2c–4c, and they represent the majority of the intermediate ploidies. For these reasons we prefer to apply the sum of intermediate ploidies rather than the subdiploidy alone in order to consider the amount of injured myocytes.

Another relevant point is the relationship between the donor age and the sum of intermediate ploidies. Our results, even if obtained in a small number of cases, indicate that age matching may be important in selecting the donor for the recipient.

87

When the donor age is smaller than 30 years or the age difference between the recipient and the donor is larger than 25 years, we can observe a markedly cellular injury in the allograft, i.e. a 59% of increase in the percentage of apoptotic myocytes, and a one-fold augmentation in the sum of intermediate ploidies. This phenomenon may be due to the anatomic, physiological, biochemical as well as hemodynamic differences in different age populations. These differences can be relevant in the remodelling of the heart in a way similar to that occurring during organogenesis (Takeda *et al.*, 1996) or postnatal maturation (Kajstura *et al.*, 1995).

Taking both ventricles into account, the sum of intermediate ploidies in the left ventricle is higher than that of the right one in the control group. This phenomenon reflectes the myocytes in the left ventricle have a higher frequency of DNA synthesis so the numbers of polyploid nuclei and multinucleated myocytes are larger than those of the right ventricle. In pathological hearts, the sum of intermediate ploidies of myocyte nuclei is nearly the same in both ventricles. Comparatively, the myocyte nuclei in the right ventricle undergo DNA synthesis at a higher frequency. These changes reduce the difference of nuclear DNA content between both ventricles (Beltrami *et al.*, 1997b, Yan *et al.*, 1998, 1999b).

In summary, end-stage cardiomyopathic hearts are characterised by an increase in the sum of intermediate ploidies. This phenomenon reveals slight in idiopathic dilated and ischemic hearts and reflects mainly the DNA synthesis. Whereas, the phenomenon shows straking in transplanted hearts and indicates mainly the DNA damage.

5.6. Total ploidy index and cardiomyopathies

Until now there are, at least, two equations for calculating the DNA content of myocytes. The first was used by Brodsky *et al.* (1991, 1994) in terms of the mean ploidy (MP) of myocytes.

$$MP = \frac{2\times\%2c + 4\times\%4c + 8\times\%8c + 16\times\%16c + 32\times\%32c + 64\times\%64c + 128\times\%128c}{\%2c + \%4c + \%8c + \%16c + \%32c + \%64c + \%128c}$$

For this equation, we can present it as a more mathematical form as follows:

$$MP = \frac{\sum_{n=1}^{7} 2^n \times \%2^n c}{\sum_{n=1}^{7} \%2^n c}$$

The calculated value in this equation is the sum of products of frequency of the myocyte class by the genome weight of the given class. The classes are defined according to the number of genomes, i.e. diploidy (2c: genome number 2); tetraploidy (mononucleated 4c and binucleated 2c times two: genome number 4); up to binucleated 64c times two: genome number 128. This equation has a solid biological meaning. However, the DNA content in cells increases according to a doubling way, i.e. 2, 4, 8, 16, 32 and 64. Thus, a slight change in high ploidy classes can lead to an unproportional change in the calculated value, consequently lead to an unproportional change in the distribution of frequencies of different ploidies. Therefore, this equation is very sensitive to the change in high ploidy classes, and suitable for the comparison between two groups with main changes in high ploidy classes.

The second equation is the calculation of the polyploidization factor (PF), in which the genome weights of different ploidy peaks undergo the $\log_2$ transformation (Vliegen *et al.*, 1991).

$$PF = \frac{2\times\%4c + 3\times\%8c + 4\times\%16c + 5\times\%32c + 6\times\%64c}{\%4c + \%8c + \%16c + \%32c + \%64c}$$

For this equation, we can present it as a more mathematical form as follows:

$$PF = \frac{\sum_{n=2}^{6} \log_2 2^n \times \%2^n c}{\sum_{n=2}^{6} \%2^n c}$$

This equation homogenizes the contributions of each ploidy to the whole ploidy population, thus it decreases the unproportional changes in high ploidy classes, and leads to the distributions of frequencies of different ploidies forward to the normality. Compared to the Brodsky's equation, it has a smaller calculated value.

However, both of the equations concern only for the myocytes in DNA ploidy peaks and ignore the myocytes in subdiploidy and intermediate ploidies. In fact, the myocytes in subdiploidy and intermediate ploidies exist in control hearts and increase significantly in pathological conditions. Therefore, we introduce the total ploidy index (TPI) for calculating the DNA content of myocytes by the following equation:

$$TPI = \frac{\% < 2c + 2 \times \%2c + 3 \times \%(2c - 4c) + 4 \times \%4c + 5 \times \%(4c - 8c) + 6 \times \%8c}{\% < 2c + \%2c + \%(2c - 4c) + \%4c + \%(4c - 8c) + \%8c}$$

$$\frac{+ 7 \times \%(8c - 16c) + 8 \times \%16c + 9 \times \%(16c - 32c) + 10 \times \%32c}{+ \%(8c - 16c) + \%16c + \%(16c - 32c) + \%32c}$$

$$\frac{+ 11 \times \%(32c - 64c) + 12 \times \%64c + 13 \times \%(64c - 128c) + 14 \times \%128c}{+ \%(32c - 64c) + \%64c + \%(64c - 128c) + \%128c}$$

We also can present our equation in a more mathematical form as follows:

$$TPI = \frac{\% < 2c + \sum_{n=3}^{8} \log_2 2^{(2n-3)} \times \%(2^{n-2}c - 2^{n-1}c) + 2\sum_{n-1}^{7} \log_2 2^n \times \%2^n c}{\% < 2c + \sum_{n=3}^{8} \%(2^{n-2}c - 2^{n-1}c) + \sum_{n=1}^{7} \%2^n c}$$

In this way the DNA content of myocytes is evaluated including ploidy peaks as well as intermediate ploidies. The values of TPI are between those of MP and PF, while the CV of TPI is similar to that of PF. Using this parameter we have analysed successfully the changes in DNA content of myocytes in control and cardiomyopathic hearts (Beltrami *et al.*, 1997b, Yan *et al.*, 1998, 1999b). As a global index of the changes in DNA content, the total ploidy index shows a marked increase in ischemic and dilated cardiomyopathies. Also, the total ploidy index reveals srtong correlations with the heart weight and ventricular weight. However, the total ploidy index shows no significant changes in transplanted hearts, even if there is an increase in myocytes having DNA content higher than 4c. This fact confirms that the increase in DNA content is balanced by the large amount of damaged DNA.

In summary, the total ploidy index can reflect the DNA content of myocytes including both ploidy peaks and intermediate ploidies. In idiopathic dilated and ischemic cardiomyopathies, the total ploidy index increases predominently with respect of high degree of polyploidization and multinucleation. In transplanted hearts, the total ploidy index shows no significant changes, because the increase in DNA content is balanced by the large amount of damaged DNA.

5.7. Nuclear area and cardiomyopathies

End-stage cardiomyopathic hearts are characterised by augmentation of nuclear size in both myocytes and interstitial cells. Meanwhile, the coefficient of variation of average nuclear area (CVANA) decreases in the interstitial cell population and increases in the myocyte population, when the cardiomyopathic hearts are compared to the control hearts (Yan et al., 1999a).

Changes in the nuclear area may reflect qualitative or quantitative alterations of DNA, which partially controls cell functions. The study on nuclear size and total RNA synthesis has been performed in single lumbar motoneurons isolated from the grass frog. The results show that transcription is correlated significantly with nuclear area or volume over a wide range of nuclear size. The largest nuclei have the highest mean transcriptional activity (Sato et al., 1994). A significant increase in the nuclear volume is accompanied with the increased nuclear ploidy (Martynova et al., 2002). Nuclear enlargement of cardiac cells represents the basis of cardiac cell growth in cardiomyopathic hearts. The biological significance of their growth, however, may be complex and various, depending upon different myocardial components. Although an increase in average nuclear area is found in both myocytes and interstitial cells, the coefficient of variation in average nuclear area changes in different ways in different cardiac populations. These facts may be useful in explaining that myocyte growth and interstitial cell growth play different roles in pathological conditions (Yan et al., 1999a). Also, the cardiomyocyte nuclei are in a dynamic state and nuclear hypertrophy and polyploidization may be a reversible phenomenon (Rivello et al., 2001).

5.7.1. Myocyte growth and cardiomyopathies

The changes in myocyte morphology partially represent structural remodeling of the heart. Disproportional myocyte growth is observed in pathologic concentric hypertrophy (myocyte thickening) and in eccentric dilated hypertrophy (myocyte lengthening). Alterations in myocyte shape can lead to changes in chamber geometry and wall stress (Savinova and Gerdes, 2012). Cardiac hypertrophy results from enhanced protein synthesis, sarcomeric reorganization and density, and increased cardiomyocyte size, all culminating into structural remodeling of the heart (Gladka et al., 2012). Remodeling myocytes show a typical switch between the embryonic and classical features of apoptosis and/or hypertrophy representing a signal of death (apoptosis) and a signal of life (hypertrophy) (Ferrari et al., 2009). Subcellular remodeling during the process of cardiac remodeling plays a major role in the development of cardiac dysfunction in congestive heart failure (Babick and Dhalla, 2007).

In end-stage ischemic cardiomyopathy, myocyte loss accounts for 28% and 30% in the left and right ventricles (Beltrami et al., 1994). In idiopathic dilated cardiomyopathy, coronary blood flow is markedly impaired (Parodi et al., 1993). This defect may result in diffuse myocardial ischemia, leading to foci of myocytolytic

92

necrosis and scattered myocyte death (Unverferth et al., 1986; Roberts et al., 1987; Beltrami et al., 1995). After cardiac transplantation, the rejection leads to multiple focal sites of myocyte necrosis across the ventricular wall (Pomerance and Stovin, 1985; Johnson et al., 1989; Rowan and Billingham, 1990; Winters, 1991; Graham, 1992; Tazelaar and Edwands, 1992; Symmans et al., 1994).

Myocyte death results in a reactive hypertrophic response of the overloaded remaining cells (Ginzton et al., 1989; Pfeffer and Braunwald, 1990; Anversa et al., 1990c, 1993). Such a condition consistently has been found in the human failing heart (Astorri et al., 1971, 1977; Gerdes et al., 1992; Beltrami et al., 1994, 1995, 2001). The mechanisms of adaptive growth of myocyte nuclei involve simple nuclear hypertrophy, polyploidization and multinucleation.

Significant nuclear hypertrophy is found in each DNA ploidy class, not only in ploidy peaks but also in intermediate ploidies. Nuclear hypertrophy shows the adaptive growth of myocyte nuclei in rats during growth and cardiac hypertrophy (Gerdes et al., 1991, 1994). The increment in nuclear area may be related to reorganisation of the related amount of extended (euchromatin) and condensed (heterochromatin) chromatin.

However, simple nuclear hypertrophy cannot be resolved with enlarged myocyte volume. The ability of a myocyte to become hypertrophic is determined by its capacity to increase its DNA content (Vliegen et al., 1990). Human cardiac myocytes can increase DNA content by polyploidization and multinucleation. In cardiomyopathies, myocyte nuclei show an increase in DNA content predominantly as a result of polyploidization. Diploid myocyte nuclei decrease and polyploid myocyte nuclei increase. The highest ploidy classes appear higher than 16c. The total ploidy index increases by 60% in ischemic cardiomyopathy and more than 70% in idiopathic dilated cardiomyopathy compared to the control hearts (Beltrami et al., 1977b). Therefore, the nuclear area of myocytes enlarges with the augmentation of nuclear DNA content. In this way, the enlargement of nuclear size becomes very impressive in myocytes. Furthermore, the increment in the degree of multinucleation enhances the DNA content and nuclear area per myocyte (Vliegen *et al.,* 1990; Beltrami *et al.,* 1997b, Yan *et al.,* 1998, 1999b).

In view of the relationship with nuclear size and DNA content of myocytes, a slight overlap of myocyte nuclear area is presented between adjacent DNA ploidy classes as well as between DNA ploidy peaks (Yan *et al.,* 1999s). However, this overlap occurrs in less than 5% of nuclei. At this stage, we could not explain this phenomenon in great detail.

5.7.2. Interstitial cell growth and cardiomyopathies

The myocardial interstitium is not a passive entity, but rather a complex and dynamic microenvironment. The structural and signaling system in the myocardium is highly organized and orchestrated, whereby small disruptions in composition, spatial relationships, or content can lead to altered myocardial systolic and/or diastolic performance. These changes in extracellular matrix structure and function are important in the progression to heart failure in pressure overload hypertrophy, dilated cardiomyopathy, and ischemic heart disease (Hutchinson et al., 2010; Eckhouse and Spinale, 2012).

The present study shows that interstitial cells have diploid nuclei. Only rare interstitial cells have nuclei with 2c–4c or 4c DNA content. It is not found that interstitial cells have nuclear DNA content higher than 4c. We consider nuclear growth of interstitial cells to be associated with simple nuclear hypertrophy rather than polyploidization. The nuclear area of interstitial cells increases without incremental increases in nuclear DNA content, so the coefficient of variation in average nuclear area decreases in both ventricles. These features reflect the homogeneity of interstitial cell growth resulting from reactive enlargement of their nuclei (Yan *et al.,* 1999a).

In previous work we quantitatively showed that collagen accumulation comprises an average of 28% and 13% of left and right ventricular myocardium in ischemic

94

cardiomyopathy (Beltrami *et al.*, 1994). Corresponding collagen accumulation occupies approximately 20% of each ventricle in idiopathic dilated cardiomyopathy (Beltrami *et al.*, 1995). Transplanted hearts show an approximately two-fold increase in the mean myocardial collagen content compared with normal hearts (van Suylenet *et al.*, 1996). The current result, nuclear enlargement of interstitial cells, can explain the activation of those cells in end-stage cardiomyopathies.

Cleutjens *et al.* showed that the increase in procollagen mRNA is associated with an increase in collagen protein deposition in both infarcted and non-infarcted areas (Cleutjens *et al.*, 1995). On the one hand, reactive fibrosis forms a scar that prevents further dilatation and rupture of the infarcted wall (Cannon *et al.*, 1983; Caulfield and Wolkowicz, 1990). On the other hand, collagen accumulation in non-infarcted area is associated with disturbances in the conducting system and increased myocardial stiffness. Progressing fibrosis leads to a reduction in the myocardial function and finally causes heart failure (Michel *et al.*, 1988; van der Laarse *et al.*, 1989b; Litwin *et al.*, 1991; Voldes *et al.*, 1993).

In summary, the current results demonstrate that nuclear size can be used as an indicator for assessing functional alterations of different cardiac cell populations in heart disease. Augmentation of nuclear size follows two ways: one is without an increase in DNA content and the other one by an increment in DNA content. In the first way, nuclear size enlarges to a limited extent. In the second, the augmentation of nuclear size can become very impressive. In end-stage cardiomyopathies, nuclear growth of myocytes and interstitial cells may be due to different mechanisms. The enlargement of nuclear area of myocytes represents a complex process including simple nuclear hypertrophy, polyploidization and multinucleation. Myocyte growth accounts for the response of myocyte death. The main pattern of nuclear growth of interstitial cells is nuclear hypertrophy without an increase in DNA content. Activated fibroblasts contribute to remodelling impaired myocardium, but progressing fibrosis may result in the reduction in myocardial function and finally cause heart failure.

5.8. Myocyte mitosis and cardiomyopathies

Several studies in humans (Beltrami *et al.*, 1994, 1995) and in animals (Capasso *et al.*, 1990; Li *et al.*, 1993; Kajstura *et al.*, 1994, 1995) have demonstrated that cellular loss of myocytes is a consistent finding of cardiac failure from various aetiologies. Myocyte cell loss accompanies the evolution of different myopathies and appears to precede the impairment in ventricular pump function (Olivetti *et al.*, 1994a, 1994b). Cell death, whether diffuse or segmental in distribution, results in mural thinning, cavitary dilation, depressed ventricular performance and a significant increase in diastolic wall stress (McKay *et al.*, 1986; Warren *et al.*, 1988; Olivetti *et al.*, 1990, 1991; Anversa *et al.*, 1992). Additionally, the transplanted hearts have to adapt to the functional demands of the host. Thus, reactive growth processes in the myocardium are initiated by the overloads on the remaining viable myocytes.

Regeneration in myocytes is identified by ultrastructural and light microscopic evidences showing cytoplasmic dedifferentiation and nuclear mitosis. Myocyte dedifferentiation has been detailed by McMahon and Ratliff (1990). Myocyte mitosis has been presented in previous works (Kazantseva and Babaev, 1977; Anversa *et al.*, 1990b; Kupper, 1991; Reiss *et al.*, 1993, 1994; Quaini *et al.*, 1994; Beltrami *et al.*, 1997a) and is further supported by the present quantitative analysis.

Kajstura *et al.* reported their quantitative results obtained by confocal microscope. In control human hearts, 14 mitoses are found in million myocytes. A nearly 10-fold increase in this parameter is measured in end-stage ischemic heart disease (152 myocytes per million) and in idiopathic dilated cardiomyopathy (131 myocytes per million). Because the left ventricle contains 5.8×10^9 myocytes, these mitotic indices imply that 81.2×10^3, 882×10^3 and 760×10^3 myocytes are in mitosis in the entire ventricular myocardium of control hearts and hearts affected by ischemic and idiopathic dilated cardiomyopathy, respectively. Additionally, mitosis lasts less than one hour, suggesting that large number of myocytes can be formed in the nonpathological and pathological heart with time. Evidence of cytokinesis in myocytes is obtained, providing unequivocal proof of myocyte proliferation (Kajstura et al., 1998). Also, our another study on the infarcted hearts showed that Ki-67 expression was detected in 4 percent of myocyte nuclei in the regions adjacent to the infarcts and in 1 percent of those in regions distant from the infarcts. The reentry of myocytes into the cell cycle resulted in mitotic indexes of 0.08% and 0.03%, respectively, in the zones adjacent to and distant from the infarcts. The formation of the mitotic spindles, contractile rings, karyokinesis, and cytokinesis were identified as characteristic of cell division, and demonstrated that the regeneration of myocytes may be a critical component of the increase in muscle mass of the myocardium (Beltrami et al.,2001).

Importantly, the capacity of myocytes ongoing nuclear mitosis shows strongly time-dependent in cardiac allografts. Within six months after heart transplantation, the occurrence and the frequency of myocyte mitosis are prominent. The reactive growth of myocytes is started as an answer to the rejection injury and to the increased functional demands associated with variables of the host. However, after six months, the occurrence of myocyte mitosis reduces sharply. This phenomenon may indicate the limited possibility of myocytes to undergo mitotic division. Moreover, we observed a lower frequency of myocyte mitosis in the cases whose donor age is smaller than 30 years or the age difference between the recipient and the donor is higher than 25 years. This may be another support to the importance for age matching in cardiac transplantation (Yan et al., 1998, 1999b).

Tissue homeostasis and regenerative capacity are nowadays considered to be related to the stem cell pool present in every tissue (Beltrami et al., 2011). The integration of carbon-14 into DNA, which established the age of cardiomyocytes in humans, showed cardiomyocytes renewal with a gradual decrease from 1% turning

97

over annually at the age of 25 to 0.45% at the age of 75 (Bergmann *et al.*, 2009). Cellular senescence can lead to irreversible growth arrest, alterations of the gene expression profile, epigenetic modifications, and an altered secretome (Beltrami *et al.*, 2012). However, functional human cardiac stem cells (hCSCs) persist in the decompensated heart, and resent study first demonstrated that dysfunctional telomeres in hCSCs can serve as biomarkers of aging and heart failure (Cesselli *et al.*, 2011). Therefore, stem cell senescence and regeneration play profound roles on the heart in both physiological and pathological circumstances.

In summary, the quantitative measurements indicate that nuclear mitoses of mtocytes appear unequivocally in control adult human hearts and increase in pathological hearts. This phenomenon is predominant in transplanted hearts, but the frequency of myocyte mitosis decrease sharply after six months of cardiac transplantation.

5.9. Nuclear DNA ploidy patterns of cardiomyocytes

The present results demonstrate the variety of nuclear DNA ploidy patterns in cardiomyocytes. The multinucleated myocytes with nuclei in different DNA ploidies are implicated of the heterogeneity of nuclear DNA ploidy patterns, which increases significantly in cardiomyopathic conditions.

5.9.1. Variety of nuclear DNA ploidy patterns in cardiomyocytes

Twelve nuclear DNA ploidy patterns are found in mononucleated myocytes (from <2c to 64c). The DNA content of myocyte nuclei is not higher than 8c in control hearts. However, the DNA content of myocyte nuclei appear remarkably high up to 64c in pathological hearts. Polyploidization results from nuclear DNA replication without karyokinesis so that myocytes can undergo DNA synthesis reaching to higher DNA ploidy.

According to the number of DNA ploidy patterns in mononucleated myocytes, theoretically, there might be 66 ploidy patterns in binucleated myocytes ($12\times11/2$), 220 ploidy patterns in trinucleated myocytes ($12\times11\times10/(3\times2)$), 495 ploidy patterns in tetranucleated myocytes ($12\times11\times10\times9/(4\times3\times2)$) and 792 ploidy patterns in pentanucleated myocytes ($12\times11\times10\times9\times8/(5\times4\times3\times2)$). In the preliminary observation, 89% of DNA ploidy patterns have been found in binucleated myocytes because of the major frequency and less combinations. Nevertheless, 52% and 29% of DNA ploidy patterns have been found in trinucleated myocytes and tetranucleated myocytes. Only 2.5% of DNA ploidy patterns have been found in myocytes with five nuclei. It is very difficult to find all ploidy patterns in cardiomyocytes due to the small fractions of multinucleated myocytes and myocytes with very high polyploidies. However, these results suggest the variety of nuclear DNA ploidy patterns in cardiomyocytes and multinucleated myocytes may have all of possible nuclear DNA ploidy patterns in various combinations.

Multinucleated myocytes and polyploid myocytes may have larger cellular size. Thus, multinucleation and polyploidizition contribute to myocyte hypertrophy which may be the dominant growth mechanism of myocardium in its compensated stage (Quaini, 1994). It is evident that multiple templates enable a cell to multiply its transcription activity. Actually, according to the positive correlation between the mass of DNA (chromatin) and the mass of cytoplasm (and organelles, ribosomes, etc.), polyploid cells are capable of high functional activities within a short period of time (Nagl, 1990).

5.9.2. Heterogeneity of nuclear DNA ploidy patterns in multinucleated myocytes

In general, the nuclei of a multinucleated cell reveal the similar size, shape and DNA content. If the cell contains two diploid nuclei, it has four chromosome sets. Many studies show that all four sets are active and that a binucleated diploid cell does not differ in its functional characteristics (transcription and translation intensity, enzyme activity, protein and glycogen content, etc.) from a mononucleated tetraploid cell of the same type (Brodsky *et al.*, 1985). The multinucleated myocytes having nuclei in the same ploidy class indicate the identity of nuclear ploidy patterns in cardiomyocytes. These nuclei may perform the same reactions to the physiological or pathological stimuli and undergo DNA replication with or without cytokinetic mitosis synchronisticly.

On the other hand, the multinucleated myocytes with nuclei in different DNA ploidies demonstrate the heterogeneity of nuclear DNA ploidy patterns. Some nuclei may undergo continued DNA synthesis containing higher DNA content while others may be static containing lower DNA content. At present, it is difficult to explain why the nuclei in the same myocyte perform in different ways.

Importantly, the quantitative study demonstrates that pathological hearts are characterised by an increase in the percentage of myocytes with nuclei in different intermediate ploidies. Thus, the heterogeneity of nuclear DNA ploidy patterns becomes apparent in diseased conditions. As mentioned above, these nuclei may come from three ways: (i) DNA synthesis, (ii) DNA lysis and (iii) abnormal mitosis. The first two points have been discussed before (Beltrami *et al.*, 1997b, Yan *et al.*, 1998, 1999b). The last one may result from chromosomal aberrations originated from the erroneous chromosome segregation (Hinchcliffe *et al.*, 1999). As presented in Figure 24, a 64c nucleus, which would form two 32c daughter nuclei through normal mitosis, forms three daughter nuclei: one 32c nucleus and other two located in different intermediate ploidies (4c–8c) and (16c–32c). The existence of abnormal mitosis of myocytes is supported by the findings of myocytes with chromatin bridge and/or extension.

In summary, the present study demonstrates the variety and the heterogeneity of nuclear DNA ploidy patterns of cardiomyocytes. End-stage cardiomyopathic hearts are characterised by the increase in the myocytes with nuclei in different ploidies and in different intermediate ploidies.

5.10. Chromatin bridges and cardiomyopathies

During mitosis chromatids separate from one another and migrate towards opposite spindle poles. The chromosomes form daughter nuclei in telophase. Our findings confirm that chromatin bridges and extensions exist in adult human cardiomyocytes. We agree the viewpoint that the bridges arise during mitosis through faults in chromosome segregation (Wolf et al., 1996). The bridges persist and most probably elongate, when the daughter nuclei separate from each other.

In some cases, the chromatin bridges are ruptured forming chromatin extensions. Therefore, in view of the relationship of chromatin bridges and extensions, we consider that they are the same case. The extremely stender chromatin bridges may be broken as the separation of two nuclei or cut as the preparation of tissue section. In these conditions, chromatin bridges became chromatin extensions.

Furthermore, a subset of chromatin bridges contains centromeres. Centromeric heterochromatin is not affected while neighbouring euchromatic segments extend during migration of the cells away from one another, indicating that the mechanical properties of euchromatin and heterochromatin differ. Heterochromatin-specific proteins may bring about these differences (Saunders et al., 1993; Nicol and Jeppesen, 1994; Wreggett et al., 1994; Starr et al., 1997). Less subtle manipulation of DNA by experimental mechanical interference stretches also the centromeric heterochromatin (Haaf and Ward, 1994). No reports concern whether DNA replication occurs within cytoplasmic chromatin strands.

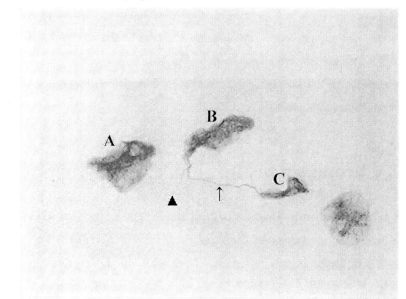

Figure 23 Myocyte with chromatin bridge and string isolated from a idiopathic dilated heart. Nuclei A, B and C have DNA content of 32c, 16c32c and 4c8c, respectively. Nuclei B and C are connected by a chromatin bridge about 50 microns (arrow). A chromatin string about 36 microns (arrowhead) initiates from Nucleus B towards Nucleus A. (Feulgen stain, ×40).

Several hypotheses concern the induction of chromatin bridges. (1) The chromatin bridges account for sister chromatid pairing in late G2/mitosis, i.e. 'conservative pairing' between complementary DNA strands belong to both sister chromatids. In this situation, the relationship between chromatin bridges exists without fragments in ana-telophase and chromasomal aberrations (Rizzoni *et al.,* 1993; Botta and Gustavino, 1997). (2) Internuclear chromatin bridges are formed by nuclear rotation. The different modalities of nuclear rotation relate to equatorial (stationary nuclei), peripheral (nuclei rotating in opposite direction) or oblique (nuclei rotating in the same direction) dispositions of chromatin bridges. Moreover, the entire nucleus can rotate. The independence of the bridge arrangements from the cell cycle phases (G1, S, G2) suggests that the nuclear rotation is probably not due to exchange of

o

substances, between the active chromatin and the cytoplasm (Barni and Scherini, 1991). (3) The existence of chromatin bridges can serve as a morphological marker of a highly mobile cell type (Wolf *et al.*, 1996). (4) The formation of chromatin bridges represents chromosomal aberrations. Some chemicals have a clastogenic activity on the DNA, such as adriamycin (Dulout and Olivero, 1984), 3'-azido-2',3'-dideoxythymidine (Olivero and Porier, 1993), bleomycin (Barni *et al.*, 1992), 2,4-diamino-6-hydroxypyrimidine (Chen *et al.*, 1994), methylmercury chloride (Tournamille *et al.*, 1982), mitomycin C (Dulout and Olivero, 1984), platinol (Katoh *et al.*, 1990), triethylenemelamine (Dulout *et al.*, 1980), trimethylpsoralen (TMP) + UVA (Rizzoni *et al*, 1993; Botta and Gustavino, 1997) and so on. There are several types of karyological damage including micronuclei, internuclear chromatin bridges and mitotic chromosome bridges. Silver nanoparticles could penetrate plant system and may impair stages of cell division causing chromatin bridge, stickiness, disturbed metaphase, multiple chromosomal breaks and cell disintegration (Kumari et al., 2009). (5) Chromatin bridges at anaphase result from mutations in lodestar, a Drosophila gene encoding a putative nucleoside triphosphate-binding protein (Girdham and Glover, 1991). (6) The chromatin bridges can be resulted from an erroneous chromosome segregation, which can partially be explained by the chromosome stickiness, telomere shortening, the exchange-type aberrations and microtubule modification (Zimmerman *et al.*, 1999; Gisselsson and Höglund 2005; Fenech 2006; Tusell *et al.*, 2010; O'Sullivan *et al.*, 2002). The abnormality of centrosome can lead directly to aneuploidy and genomic instability through the formation of multipolar mitotic spindles (Hinchcliffe *et al.*, 1999; Genescà *et al.*, 2011). At present, not clear are the real reasons for the induction of chromatin bridges in cardiomyocytes.

We infer that there are three outcomes of the daughter myocytes with chromosomal aberrations including chromatin bridges and extensions. (i) Slight alteration in nuclear DNA leads to the living myocytes with normal function. (ii) Moderate alteration in nuclear DNA results in the living myocytes cannot perform

103

normal contraction. The reduction of ventricular function stimulates reactive hypertrophy of the living myocytes. Consequently, the cardiac function is improved when the hypertrophic myocytes have higher contractive ability; otherwise the deterioration of cardiac function continues because of the hypertrophic myocytes without normal function. (iii) Severe alteration in nuclear DNA induces myocyte apoptosis (Levkau et al., 2008). In this case, the mitosis of differentiated myocytes may be accompanied by nuclear DNA damage leading to cellular death (Kazantseva and Babaev, 1977; Lane, 1992; Latif et al., 2000; Urbanek et al., 2005).

Recent studies reveal pathways related to the formation of chromatin bridges. Chromosomal instability occurs early in the development of cancer and may represent an important step in promoting the multiple genetic changes required for the initiation and/or progression of the disease (Tusell et al., 2010). Telomere dysfunction contributes to chromosome instability through end-to-end chromosome fusions entering breakage-fusion-bridge (BFB) cycles. Resolution of chromatin bridge intermediates is likely to contribute greatly to the generation of segmental chromosome amplification events, unbalanced chromosome rearrangements, and whole chromosome aneuploidy (Genescà et al., 2011). The putative chromatin remodeling enzyme Plk1-interacting checkpoint helicase (PICH) was discovered as an interaction partner and substrate of the mitotic kinase Plk1. The interference with PICH function results in chromatin bridge formation and micronucleation (Kaulich et al., 2012). Tumor-associated microtubule-associated protein (TMAP), also known as cytoskeleton associated protein 2 (CKAP2), is a novel mitotic spindle-associated protein which is frequently up-regulated in various malignances (Hong et al., 2009). Additionally, a regulatory subunit of protein phosphatase 2A (Tap46) plays role on sister chromatid segregation as its silencing in tobacco (Nicotiana tabacum) BY-2 cells can cause chromatin bridge formation at anaphase (Ahn et al., 2011).

There are several types of karyological damage have been found in this study, such as irregular nuclear shape (Nuclei B and C in Fig. 23), nuclear vacuole (the small nucleus in Panels B and D in Fig. 21), micronucleus (Panel I in Fig. 21) and so

104

on. Because the adult left ventricle contains an average of 5.2 billion myocyte nuclei (Olivetti *et al.*, 1991), it is not ignored the existence of the myocytes with chromatin bridge and/or extension. These myocytes increase significantly in pathological hearts, especially in idiopathic dilated cardiomyopathy (more than 600 myocytes per million). Thus, the chromosomal aberrartion may be one of the reasons for myocyte death and heart failure.

In summary, end-stage cardiomyopathic hearts are characterised by the increase in myocytes with chromatin bridge and/or extension. These findings suggest that the chromosomal aberrartion may be one of the reasons for myocyte dysfunction and myocyte death leading to cardiac deterioration.

6. ACKNOWLEDGEMENTS

My Ph.D. study was performed at the Department of Pathology, University of Udine. I would like to thank many people who have helped me during the study, including professors, doctors, technicians and others.

I am very greatful to *Centro di Riferimento Oncologico, Istituto Nazionale di Ricovero e Carattera Scientifico, Aviano, Italy* for the financial support.

I also wish to extend my gratitude to my family, my hudsband and my son, as well as my relatives who have been giving me persistent supports.

7. REFFERENCES

Adler CP (1986). Histochemically determinable changes in cardiac insufficiency and their functional significance. *Basic Res Cardiol* 81(suppl 1): 179–192.

Adler CP (1991). Polyploidization and augmentation of heart muscle cells during normal cardiac growth and in cardiac hypertrophy. *In: The development and regeneration potential of cardiac muscle.* Edited by Oberpriller JO, Mauro A. New York; Harwood Academic Publishers, pp: 227–252.

Adler CP, Costabel U (1975). Post mortem investigations of human hearts. *Virchows Arch (B)* 16: 343–355.

Adler CP, Sandritter W (1971). Polyploidization of the myocardium in cardiac hypertrophy. *Verh Dtsch Ges Inn Med* 77: 1252–1256.

Ahn CS, Han JA, Lee HS, Lee S, Pai HS (2011). The PP2A regulatory subunit Tap46, a component of the TOR signaling pathway, modulates growth and metabolism in plants. *Plant Cell* 23: 185–209.

Antipanova EM, Erokhina IL, Rumiantsev PP (1987). Levels of DNA and sex chromatin bodies in the myocyte nuclei of different sections of human hearts. *Tsitologiia* 29: 782–787.

Anversa P, Beghi C, Kikkawa Y, Olivetti G (1985). Myocardial response to infarction in the rat: Morphometric measurement of infarct size and myocyte cellular hypertrothy. *Am J Pathol* 118: 484–492.

Anversa P, Beghi C, Kikkawa Y, Olivetti G (1986). Myocardial infarction in rats: Infarct size, myocyte hypertrophy, and capillary growth. *Circ Res* 58: 56–37.

Anversa P, Fitzpatrick D, Argani S, Capasso JM (1991). Myocyte mitotic division in the aging mammanlian rat heart. *Circ Res* 69: 1159–1164.

Anversa P, Kajstura J, Cheng W, Reiss K, Cigola E, Olivetti G (1996a). Insulin-like growth factor-1 and myocyte growth: The danger of a dogma. Part I. Postnatal myocardial development: Normal growth. *Cardiovasc Res* 32: 219–225.

Anversa P, Kajstura J, Cheng W, Reiss K, Cigola E, Olivetti G (1996b). Insulin-like growth factor-1 and myocyte growth: The danger of a dogma. Part II. Induced myocardial growth: Pathologic hypertrophy. *Cardiovasc Res* 32: 484–495.

Anversa P, Leri A, Beltrami CA, Guerra S, Kajstura J (1998). Myocyte death and growth in the failing heart. *Lab Invest* 78: 767–786.

Anversa P, Li P, Zhang X, Olivetti G, Capasso JM (1993). Ischemic myocardial injury and ventricular remodeling. *Cardiovasc Res* 27: 145–157.

Anversa P, Olivetti G, Leri A, Liu Y, Kajstura J (1997). Myocyte cell death and ventricular remodlling. *Curr Opin Nephrol Hypertens* 6: 169–176.

Anversa P, Palackal T, Sonnenblick EH, Olivetti G, Capasso JM (1990a). Hypertensive cardiomyopathy: Myocyte nuclear hyperplasia in the mammalian heart. *J Clin Invest* 85: 994–997.

Anversa P, Palackal T, Sonnenblick EH, Olivetti G, Meggs LG, Capasso JM (1990b). Myocyte cell loss and myocyte cellular hyperplasia in the hypertrophied aging rat heart. *Circ Res* 67: 871–885.

Anversa P, Sonnenblick EH (1990c). Ischemic cardiomyopathy: pathophysiologic mechanisms. *Prog Cardiovasc Dis* 33: 49–70.

Anversa P, Zhang X, Li P, Capasso JM (1992). Chronic coronary artery constriction leads to moderate myocyte loss and left ventricular dysfunction and failure in rats. *J Clin Invest* 89: 618–629.

Arbustini E, Pozzi R, Grasso M, Gavazzi A, Diegoli M, Bramerio M, Graziano G, Campana C, Angoli L, DeServi S, Martinelli L, Goggi C, Vigano M, Specchia G (1991). Pathologic substrates and clinical correlates of coronary artery disease and chronic congestive heart failure requiring cardiac transplantation. *Coron Artery Dis* 2: 605–612.

Arefyeva AM, Mares V, Ostadal B, Brodsky WY (1985). A cytophotometric and karyometric study of the cardiac muscle cells of young rats exposed to intermittent high altitude hypoxia. *Physiol Bohemoslov* 34: 94–96.

Astorri E, Bolognesi R, Colla B, Chizzola A, Visioli O (1977). Left ventricular hypertrophy: a cytometric study on 42 human hearts. *J Mol Cell Cardiol* 9: 763–775

Astorri E, Chizzola A, Visioli O, Anversa P, Olivetti G, Vitali-Mazza L (1971). Right ventricular hypertrophy: a cytometric study on 55 human hearts. *J Mol Cell Cardiol* 2: 99–110.

Babick AP, Dhalla NS (2007). Role of subcellular remodeling in cardiac dysfunction due to congestive heart failure. *Med Princ Pract.* 16: 81–89.

Bardales RH, Shea Hailey L, Xie SS, Schaefer RF, Hsu S (1996). In situ apoptosis assay for the detection of early acute myocardial infarction. *Am J Pathol* 149: 821–829.

Barni S, Porcelli F, Scherini E, Spadari S (1992). Induction of Karyological damage by bleomycin in polyploidizing rabbit hepatocytes. *Anticancer Res* 12: 521–528.

Barni S, Scherini E (1991). Possible patterns of nuclear rotation in binucleate hepatocytes in vivo: static examination with fluorescence and electron microscope. *In Vivo* 5: 167–170.

Baroldi G, Falza G, Lampertico P (1967). The nuclear patterns of the cardiac muscle fiber. *Cardiologia* 51: 109–123.

Beltrami CA, Della Mea V, Finato N, Rocco M (1996). Computer-assisted morphometric analysis of the heart. *Anal Quant Cytol Histol* 18: 129–136.

Beltrami CA, Di Loreto C, Finato N, Rocco M, Artico D, Cigola E, Gambert SR, Olivetti G, Kajstura J, Anversa P (1997a). Proliferating cell nuclear antigen (PCNA), DNA synthesis and Mitosis in myocytes following cardiac transplantation in man. *J Mol Cell Cardiol* 29: 2789–2802.

Beltrami CA, Di Loreti C, Finato N, Yan SM (1997b). DNA content in end-stage heart failure. *Adv Clin Path* 1: 59–73.

Beltrami CA, Finato N, Rocco M, Ferugulio GA, Puricelli C, Cigola E, Quaini F, Sonnenblick EH, Olivetti G, Anversa P (1994). Structural basis of end-stage failure in ischemic cardiomyopathy in humans. *Circulation* 89: 151–163.

Beltrami CA, Finato N, Rocco M, Feruglio GA, Puricelli C, Cigola E, Sonnenblick EH, Olivetti G, Anversa (1995). The cellular basis of dilated cardiomyopathy in human. *J Mol Cell Cardiol* 27: 291–305.

Beltrami AP, Cesselli D, Beltrami CA (2011). At the stem of youth and health. *Pharmacol Ther* 129: 3–20.

Beltrami AP, Cesselli D, Beltrami CA (2012). Stem cell senescence and regenerative paradigms. *Clin Pharmacol Ther* 91: 21–29.

Beltrami AP, Urbanek K, Kajstura J, Yan SM, Finato N, Bussani R, Nadal-Ginard B, Silvestri F, Leri A, Beltrami CA, Anversa P (2001). Evidence that human cardiac myocytes divide after myocardial infarction. *N Engl J Med* 344:1750–1757.

Bergmann O, Bhardwaj RD, Bernard S, Zdunek S, Barnabé-Heider F, Walsh S, Zupicich J, Alkass K, Buchholz BA, Druid H, Jovinge S, Frisén J (2009). Evidence for cardiomyocyte renewal in humans. *Science* 324: 98–102.

Böcking A, Striepecke E, Auer H, Füzesi L (1994). Static DNA cytometry: Biological background, technique and diagnostic interpretation. *In: Compendium on the Computerized Cytology and Histology Laboratory*. Edited by Wied GL, Bartels PH, Rosenthal DL, Schenck U. Chicago, Tutorials of Cytology, pp 107–128.

Bogenrann E, Eppenberger HM (1980). DNA-synthesis and polyploidization of chicken heart muscle cells in mass cultures. *J Mol Cell Cardiol* 12: 17–27.

Botta R, Gustavino B (1997). Relationship between chromatin bridges in anaphase and chromosomal aberrations induced by TMP + UVA in CHO cells. *Mutat Res* 374: 253–259.

Brodskii Via, Vasil'eva IA, Panova NV, Sarkisvo DS, Aref'eva AM (1989). The ploidy variability of human cardiomyocytes. *Biull Eksp Biol Med* 108: 746–748.

Brodsky VY, Sarkisov DS, Arefyeva AM, Panova NW, Gvasava IG (1994). Polyploidy in cardiac myocytes of normal and hypertrophic human hearts; range of values. *Virchows Archiv* 424: 429–435.

Brodsky VY, Carlson BM, Arefieva AM, Vacilieva IA (1988). Polyploidization of transplanted cardiac myocytes. *Cell Differ Dev* 25: 177–183.

Brodsky VY, Chernyaev AL, Vasilyeva IA (1991). Variability of the cardiomyocyte ploidy in normal human hearts. *Virchows Archiv B Cell Pathol* 61: 289–294.

Brodsky VY, Karlson BM, Arefyeva AM (1986). Polyploidization of cardiac myocytes as a programmed event of ontogenesis. *Ontofenez* 17: 138–145.

Brodsky VY, Sarkisov DS, Arefyeva AM, Panova NW (1993). DNA and protein relations in cardiomyocytes. Growth reserve in cardiac muscle. *Eur J Histochem* 37: 199–206.

Brodsky VY, Arefyeva AM, Uryvaeva IV (1980). Mitotic polyploidization of mouse heart myocytes during the first postnatal week. *Cell Tissue Res* 210: 133–144.

Brodsky VY, Tsirekidze NN, Arefyeva AM (1985). Mitotic-cyclin and cycle-independent growth of cardiomyocytes. *J Mol Cell Cardiol* 17: 445–455.

Brouwer WP, van Dijk SJ, Stienen GJ, van Rossum AC, van der Velden J, Germans T (2011). The development of familial hypertrophic cardiomyopathy: from mutation to bedside. *Eur J Clin Invest* 41: 568–578.

Buerke M, Murohara T, Skurk S, Nuss C, Tomaselli K, Lefer AM (1995). Cardioprotective effect of insulin-like growth factor I in myocardial ischemia followed by reperfusion. *Proc Natl Acad Sci USA* 92: 8031–8035.

Buja LM, Willerson JT (1987). The role of coronary artery lesions in ischemic heart disease: Insight from resent clinical copathologic, coronary arteriographic, and experimental studies. *Hum Pathol* 18: 451–461.

Cannon RO, Butany JW, McManus BM, Speir E, Kravitz AB, Bolli R, Ferrans VJ (1983), Early degradation of collagen after acute myocardial infarction in the rat. *Am J Cardiol* 52: 390–395.

Capasso JM, Bruno S, Cheng W, Li P, Rodgers R, Darzynkiewicz Z, Anversa P (1992a). Ventricular loading is coupled with DNA synthesis in adult cardiac myocytes after acute and chronic myocardial infarction in rats. *Circ Res* 71: 1379–1389.

Capasso JM, Li p, Zhang X, Anversa P (1992b). Heterogeneity of ventricular remodeling after acute myocardial infarction in rats. *Am J Physiol* 262: H486–H495.

Capasso JM, Li P, Anversa P (1993). Cytosolic calcium transients in myocytes isolated from rats with ischemic heart failure. *Am J Physiol* 265: H1953–H1964.

Capasso JM, Palackal T, Olivetti G, Anversa P (1990). Left ventrivular failure induced by long-term hypertension in rats. *Circ Res* 66: 1400–1412.

Carey FA (1994). Measurement of nuclear DNA content in histological and cytological specimens: principles and applications. *J Pathol* 172: 307–312.

Carlquist JF, Greenwood JH, Hammond EH, Anderson JL (1993). Phenotype and serine esterase production of human cardiac allograft-infiltrating lymphocytes. *Heart Lung Transplant* 12: 748–55.

Cesselli D, Beltrami AP, D'Aurizio F, Marcon P, Bergamin N, Toffoletto B, Pandolfi M, Puppato E, Marino L, Signore S, Livi U, Verardo R, Piazza S, Marchionni L, Fiorini C, Schneider C, Hosoda T, Rota M, Kajstura J, Anversa P, Beltrami CA, Leri A (2011). Effects of age and heart failure on human cardiac stem cell function. *Am J Pathol* 179: 349–366.

Caulfield JB, Wolkowicz PE (1990). Mechanisms for cardial dilatation. *Heart Failure* 6: 138–150.

Chen X, Reynolds ER, Ranganayakulu G, O'Donnell JM (1994). A maternal product of the Punch locus of Drosophila melanogaster is required for precellular blastoderm nuclear divisions. *J Cell Sci* 107: 3501–3513.

Cheng W, Li P, Kajstura J, Li B, Reiss K, Liu Y, Clark WA, Krajewski S, Reed JC, Olivetti G, Anversa P (1996). Stretch-induced programmed myocyte cell death. *J Clin Invest* 74: 86–107.

Cheng W, Reiss K, Kajetura J, Kowal K, Quaini F, Anversa P (1995). Down-regulation of the IGF-1 system parallels the attenuation in the proliferative capacity of rat ventrivular myocytes during postnatal development. *Lab Invest* 72: 646–655.

Chien KR, Knowlton KU, Zhu N, Chien S (1991). Regulation of cardiac gene expression during myocardial growth and hypertrophy: Molecular studies of an adaptive physiologic response. *FASEB J* 55: 3037–3046.

Claycomb WC, Moses RL (1985). Culture of atrial and ventricular cardiac muscle cells from adult squirrel monkey saimiri sciureus. *Exp Cell Res* 161: 95–100.

Claycomb WC, Moses RL (1988). Growth factor and TPA stimulate DNA synthesis and alter the morphology of cultured terminally differentiated adult rat cardiac muscle cells. *Dev Biol* 127: 257–265.

Cleutjens JPM, Verluyten MJA, Smits JFM, Daemen MJAP (1995). Collagen remodeling after myocardial infarction in the rat heart. *Am J Pathol* 147: 325–338.

Coen H, Pauwels M, Roels F (1992). The rat liver cell nuclear imprint as a standard for DNA measurements. *Analyt Cell Pathol* 4: 273–285.

Darzynkiewicz Z, Bruno S, Del Bino G, Gorczyca W, Hotz MA, Lassota P, Traganos F (1992). Features of apoptotic cells measured by flow cytometry. *Cytometry* 13: 795–808.

Demetris AJ, Murase N, Ye Q, Galvao FH, Richert C, Saad R, Pham S, Duquesnoy RJ, Zeevi A, Fung JJ, Starzl TE (1997). Analysis of chronic rejection and obliterative arteriopathy. Possible contributions of donor antigen-presenting cells and lymphatic disruption. *Am J Pathol* 150: 563–578.

Di Loreto C, Artico D, Finato N, Beltrami CA (1995). Proliferative activity of myocytes in transplanted haerts investigated using BrdU. *Annals New York Academy of Sciences* 752: 111–114.

Dulout FN, Larramendy ML, Olivero OA (1980). Enhancement by caffeine of the frequency of anaphase-telophase chromatin bridges induced by triethylenemelamine (TEM). *Experientia* 36: 346–347.

Dulout FN, Olivero OA (1984). Anaphastelophase analysis of chromosomal damage induced by chemicals. *Environ Mutagen* 6: 299–310.

Dorn GW 2nd (2010). Mechanisms of non-apoptotic programmed cell death in diabetes and heart failure. *Cell Cycle* 9: 3442–3448.

Ebert L, Pfitzer P (1977). Nuclear DNA of myocardial cells in the periphery of infarctions and scars. *Virchows Arch B Cell Pathol* 24: 209–217.

Eckhouse SR, Spinale FG (2012). Changes in the myocardial interstitium and contribution to the progression of heart failure. *Heart Fail Clin* 8: 7–20.

Erokhina IL, Selivanova GV, Vlasova TD, Emel'ianova OI (1995). The DNA and protein content of atrial cardiomyocytes and the size and ultrastructure of the cardiomyocytes in children with congenital heart defects. *Tsitologiia* 37: 101–108.

Erokhina IL, Selivanova GV, Vlasova TD, Komarova NI, Emeljanova OI, Soroka VV (1992). Ultrastracture and biosynthetic activity of polyploid atrial myocytes in patients with mitral vavle disease. *Acta Histochem Suppl* 42: 293–299.

Fenech M (2006). Cytokinesis-block micronucleus assay evolves into a "cytome" assay of chromosomal instability, mitotic dysfunction and cell death. *Mutat Res* 600: 58–66.

Ferrari R, Ceconi C, Campo G, Cangiano E, Cavazza C, Secchiero P, Tavazzi L (2009). Mechanisms of remodelling: a question of life (stem cell production) and death (myocyte apoptosis). *Circ J* 73: 1973–1982.

Frenzel H, Schwartzkopff B, Holtermann W, Schnurch HG, Novi A, Hort W (1988). Regression of cardiac hypertrophy: morphometric and biochemical studies in rat heart after swimming training. *J Mol Cell Cardiol* 20: 737–751.

Frisch B, Lewis SM, Sherman D (1975). The ultrastructure of dyserythropoiesis in aplastic anaemia. *Br J Haematol* 29: 545–552.

Genescà A, Pampalona J, Frías C, Domínguez D, Tusell L (2011). Role of telomere dysfunction in genetic intratumor diversity. *Adv Cancer Res* 112: 11–41.

Gerdes AM, Kellerman SE, Moore JA, Muffly KE, Clark LC, Reaves PY, Malec KB, McKeown PP, Schocken DD (1992). Stractural remodeling of cardiac myocytes in patients with ischemic cardiomyopathy. *Circulation* 86: 426–430.

Gerdes AM, Liu Z, Zimmer HG (1994). Changes in nuclear size of cardiac myocytes during the development and progression of hypertrophy in rats. *Cardioscience* 5: 203–208.

Gerdes AM, Morales MC, Handa V, Moore JA, Alvarez MR (1991). Nuclear size and DNA content in rat cardiac myocytes during growth, maturation and aging. *J Mol Cell Cardiol* 23: 833–839.

Ginzton LE, Conant R, Rodriques DM, Laks MM (1989). Functional significance of hypertrophy of the noninfarcted myocardium after myocardial infarction in humans. *Circulation* 80: 816–822.

Girdham CH, Glover DM (1991). Chromosome tangling and breakage at anaphase result from mutations in lodestar, a Drosophila gene encoding a putative nucleoside triphosphate-binding protein. *Genes Dev* 5: 1786–1799.

Gisselsson D, Höglund M (2005). Connecting mitotic instability and chromosome aberrations in cancer--can telomeres bridge the gap? *Semin Cancer Biol* 15: 13–23.

Gladka MM, da Costa Martins PA, De Windt LJ (2012). Small changes can make a big difference - microRNA regulation of cardiac hypertrophy. *J Mol Cell Cardiol* 52: 74–82.

Gottlieb RA, Burleson KO, Kloner RA, Bablor BM, Engler RL (1994). Reperfusion injury induces apoptosis in rabbit cardiomyocytes. *J Clin Invest* 94: 1621–1628.

Grabner W, Pfitzer P (1974). Number of nuclei in isolated myocardial cells of pigs. *Virchows Arch B* 15: 279–294.

Graham AR (1992). Autopsy findings in cardiac transplant patients: a 10-year experience. *Am J Clin Pathol* 97: 369–375.

Grajek S, Lesiak M, Puyda M, Zajac M, Paradowski ST, Kaczmarek E (1993). Hypertrophy or hyperplasia in cardiac muscle. Post-mortem human morphometric study. *Eur Heart J* 14: 40–47.

Grove D, Zak R, Nair KG, Aschenbrenner V (1969). Biochemical correlates or cardiac hypertrophy. IV. Observations on the cellular organization of growth during myocardial hypertrophy in the rat. *Circ Res* 25: 473–485.

Gwathmey JK, Bentivegna LA, Ransil BJ, Grossman W, Morgan JP (1993). The relationship of abnormal intracellular calcium mobilization to myocyte hypertrophy in human ventricular muocardium. *Cardiovasc Res* 27: 199–203.

Gwathmey JK, Copelas L, Makinnon R, Shoen FJ, Feldman MD, Grossman W, Morgan JP (1987). Abnormal intracellular calcium handling in myocardium from patients with end-stage heart failure. *Circ Res* 61: 70–76.

Gwathmey JK, Haijar RJ (1990). Effect of protein kinase C activation on sarcoplasmic reticulum function and apparent myofibrillar $Ca2+$ sensitivity in intact and shinned muscles from normal and diseased human myocardium. *Circ Res* 67: 744–752.

Haaf T, Ward DC (1994). Structural analysis of α-satellite DNA and centromere protein using extended chromatin and chromosomes. *Hum Mol Genet* 3: 697–709.

Hayashi S, Takamatsu T, Fujita S (1986). Cytofluorometric nuclear DNA determinations on the atrioventricular nodal cells in human hearts. *Histochemistry* 85: 111–115.

Healy MJR (1979). Outliers in clinical chemistry quality-control schemes. *Clin Chem* 25: 675–677.

Hein S, Arnon E, Kostin S, Schönburg M, Elsässer A, Polyakova V, Bauer EP, Klövekorn WP, Schaper J (2003). Progression from compensated hypertrophy to failure in the pressure-overloaded human heart: structural deterioration and compensatory mechanisms. *Circulation* 07: 984–991.

Herget GW, Neuburger M, Plagwitz R, Adler CP (1997). DNA content, ploidy level and number of nuclei in the human heart after myocardial infarction. *Cardiovasc Res* 36: 45–51.

Hinchcliffe EH, Li C, Thompson EA, Maller J, Sluder G (1999). Requirment of Cdk2-cyclin E activity for repeated centrosome reproduction on *Xenopus* egg extracts. *Science* 283: 851–854.

Hiraoka A, Kanayama Y, Yonezama T, Kitani T, Tarui S, Hashimoto PH (1983). Congenital dyserythropoietic anemia type I; a freeze-fracture and thin section electron microscopic study. *Blut* 46: 329–338.

Hong KU, Kim E, Bae CD, Park J (2009). TMAP/CKAP2 is essential for proper chromosome segregation. *Cell Cycle* 8: 314–324.

Hort W (1953). Quantitative histological examination on hypertrotric hearts. *Virchows Arch A* 323: 223–242.

Huhn KM, Palcic B, Wilson JE, McManus BM (1995). Cytometric analysis of ventricular myocyte nuclei in idiopahic dilated cardiomyopathy: a tool for evaluation of disease progression? *Eur Heart J* 16 Suppl: OP 97–99.

Hutchinson KR, Stewart JA Jr, Lucchesi PA (2010). Extracellular matrix remodeling during the progression of volume overload-induced heart failure. *J Mol Cell Cardiol* 48: 564–569.

Itoh G, Tamura J, Suzuki M, Suzuki Y, Ikeda H, Kioke M, Nomura M, Jei T, Ito K (1995). DNA fragmentation of human infarcted myocardial cells demonstrated by the nick end labelling method and DNA agarose gel electrophoresis. *Am J Pathol* 146: 1325–1331.

James TN, Martin ES, Willis PW, Lohr TO (1996). Apoptosis as a possible cause of gradual development of complete heart block and fatal arrhythmias associated with absence of the AV node, sinus node and internodal pathways. *Circulation* 93: 1424–1438.

Jean R, Dossa D, Navarro M, Rizkalla N, Lambert MF, Wagner A (1975). Congenital aplastic anemia, type I. *Arch Fr Pediatr* 32: 337–348.

Johnson DE, Gao SZ, Schroeder JS, DeCampli WM, Billingham ME (1989). The spectrum of coronary artery pathologic findings in human cardiac allografts. *J Heart Transplant* 8: 349–359.

Johnson R (1992). *Elementary statistics*. Boston, PWS-KENT Publishing Company, pp 106–110.

Joseph MC, Silvia B, Cheng W, Li P, Rodgers R, Darzynkiewicz Z, Anversa P (1992). Ventricular loading is coupled with DNA synthesis in adult cardiac myocytes after acute and chronic myocardial infarction in rats. *Circ Res* 71: 1379–1389.

Jugdutt BI (2012). Ischemia/Infarction. *Heart Fail Clin* 8: 43–51.

Kajstura J, Cheng W, Reiss K, Clark WA, Sonnenblick EH, Krajewsky S, Reed JC, Olivetti G, Anversa P (1996a). Apoptotic and necrotic myocyte cell deaths are independent contributing variables of infarct size in rats. *Lab Invest* 74: 86–107.

Kajstura J, Cheng W, Sarangarajan R, Li P, Li B, Nitahara JA, Chapnick S, Reiss K, Olivetti G, Anversa P (1996b). Necrotic and apoptotic myocyte cell death in the aging heart of Fischer 344 rats. *Am J Physiol* 271: H1215–1228.

Kajstura J, Leri A, Finato N, Di Loreto C, Beltrami CA, Anversa P (1998). Myocyte proliferation in end-stage cardiac failure in humans. *Proc Natl Acad Sci USA* 95: 8801–8805.

Kajstura J, Mansukhani M, Cheng W, Reiss K, Krajewski S, Reed JC, Quaini F, Sonnenblick EH, Anversa P (1995). Programmed cell death and the expression of the protooncogene Bcl-2 in myocyte during postnatal maturation of the heart. *Exp Cell Res* 219: 110–121.

Kajstura J, Zhang X, Reiss K, Szoke E, Li P, Lagrasta C, Cheng W, Darzynkiewicz Z, Olivetti G, Anversa P (1994). Myocyte cellular hyperplasia and myocyte cellular hypertrophy contribute to chronic ventricular remodeling in coronary artery narrowing-induced cardiomyopathy in rats. *Circ Res* 74: 383–400.

Karsner HT, Saphir O, Todd TW (1925). The state of the cardiac muscle in hypertrophy and atrophy. *Am J Pathol* 1: 351–371.

Katoh MA, Cain KT, Hughes LA, Foxworth LB, Bishop JB, Generoso WM (1990). Female-specific dominant lethal effects in mice. *Mutat Res* 230: 205–217.

Kaulich M, Cubizolles F, Nigg EA (2012). On the regulation, function, and localization of the DNA-dependent ATPase PICH. *Chromosoma* 121: 395–408.

Kawaguchi N, Kirchhof P, Fabritz L, Stypmann J, Stegger L, Flögel U, Schrader J, Fischer J, Hsieh P, Ou YL, Mehrhof F, Tiemann K, Ghanem A, Matus M, Neumann J, Heusch G, Schmid KW, Conway EM, Baba HA (2008). Survivin determines cardiac function by controlling total cardiomyocyte number. *Circulation* 117: 1583–1593.

Kawano H, Okada R, Kawano Y, Sueyoshi N, Shirai T (1994). Apoptosis in acute and chronic myocarditis. *Jpn Heart J* 35: 745–750.

Kazantseva IA, Babaev VR (1977). Mitotic division of the nuclei of the human heart myocytes after healing of myocardial infarct. *Arkh Patol* 39: 64–66.

Kazantseva IA, Babaev VR (1979). Regenerative reactions of myocardiocyte nuclei in ischemic heart disease. *Arkh Patol* 41(8): 18–23.

Kellerman S, Moore JA, Zierhut W, Zimmer HG, Campbell J, Gerdes AM (1992). Nuclear DNA content and nucleation patterns in rat cardiac myocytes from different models of cardiac hypertrophy. *J Mol Cell Cardiol* 24: 497–505.

Kirshenbaum LA, Abdellatif M, Chakraborty S, Schneider MD (1996). Human E2F-1 reactivates cell cycle progression in ventricular myocytes and represses cardiac gene transcription. *Dev Biol* 179: 402–411.

Klug MG, Soonpaa MH, Field LJ (1995). DNA synthesis and multinucleation in embryonic stem cell-derived cardiomyocytes. *Am J Physiol* 269: H1913–1921.

Korecky B, Sweet S, Rakusan K (1979). Number of nuclei in mammlian cardiac myocytes. *Can J Physiol Pharmacol* 57: 1122–1129.

Kostin S (2005). Pathways of myocyte death: implications for development of clinical laboratory biomarkers. *Adv Clin Chem* 40: 37–98.

Kranz D, Fuhrmaan I, Keim U (1975). Contribution on the physiological heart growth (Experimental autoradiographic studies in mice). *Z Mikrosk Anat Forsch* 89: 207–218.

Kumari M, Mukherjee A, Chandrasekaran N (2009). Genotoxicity of silver nanoparticles in Allium cepa. *Sci Total Environ* 407: 5243–5246.

Kung G, Konstantinidis K, Kitsis RN (2011). Programmed necrosis, not apoptosis, in the heart. *Circ Res* 108: 1017–1036.

Kupper T, Pfitzer P, Schulte D, Arnold G (1991). Pressure induced hypertrophy in the hearts of growing dwarf pigs. *Pathol Res Pract* 187: 315–323.

Lacroix B, Maddox AS (2012). Cytokinesis, ploidy and aneuploidy. *J Pathol* 226: 338–351.

Laguens RP, Cabeza Meckert PM, San Martino J, Perrone S, Favaloro R (1997). Identification of programmed cell death (apoptosis) in situ by means of specific labeling of nuclear DNA fragmentation in heart biopsy samples during acute rejection episodes. *J Heart Lung Transplant* 15: 911–918.

Lakdawala NK, Winterfield JR, Funke BH (2012). Dilated Cardiomyopathy. *Circ Arrhythm Electrophysiol* 171: 318–321.

Lane DP (1992). p53, guardian of the genome. *Nature* 358: 15–16.

Latif N, Khan MA, Birks E, O'Farrell A, Westbrook J, Dunn MJ, Yacoub MH (2000). Upregulation of the Bcl-2 family of proteins in end stage heart failure. *J Am Coll Cardiol* 35:1769–1777.

Levkau B, Schäfers M, Wohlschlaeger J, von Wnuck Lipinski K, Keul P, Hermann S, Kawaguchi N, Kirchhof P, Fabritz L, Stypmann J, Stegger L, Flögel U, Schrader J, Fischer J, Hsieh P, Ou YL, Mehrhof F, Tiemann K, Ghanem A, Matus M, Neumann J, Heusch G, Schmid KW, Conway EM, Baba HA (2008). Survivin determines cardiac function by controlling total cardiomyocyte number. *Circulation* 117:1583–1593.

Li F, Wang X, Yi XP, Gerdes AM (2004). Structural basis of ventricular remodeling: role of the myocyte. *Curr Heart Fail Rep* 1: 5–8.

Li P, Hofmann PA, Li B, Malhotra A, Cheng W, Sonnenblick EH, Meggs LG, Anversa P (1997). Myocardial infarction alters myofilament calcium sensitivity and mechanical behavior of myocytes. *Am J Physiol* 272: H360–H370.

Li P, Park C, Micheletti R, Li B, Chang W, Sonnenblick EH, Anversa P, Bianchi G (1995). Myocyte performance during evolution of myocardial infarction in rats: Effects of propionyl-L-canitine. *Am J Physiol* 268: H1702–H1713.

Li P, Zhang X, Capasso JM, Meggs LG, Sonnenblick EH, Anversa P (1993). Myocyte loss and left ventricular failure characterize the long term effects of coronary artery narrowing or renal hypertension in rats. *Cardiovasc Res* 27: 1066–1075.

Liao R, Naschimben L, Friedrich J, Gwathmey JK, Ingwall JS (1996). Decreased energy reserve in an animal model of dilated cardiomyopathy. Relationship to contractile performance. *Circ Res* 78: 893–902.

Linzbach AJ (1960). Heart failure from the point of view of quantitative anatomy. *Am J Cardiol* 5: 370–382.

Litwin SE, Litwin CM, Raya TE, Warner AL, Goldman S (1991). Contractility and stiffness of noninfacted myocardium after coronary ligation in rats. Effects of chronic angiotensin converting enzyme inhibition. *Circulation* 83: 1028–1037.

Liu Y, Cigola E, Cheng W, Kajstura J, Olivetti G, Hintze TH, Anversa P (1995). Myocyte nuclear mitotic division and programmed myocyte cell death characterize the cardiac myopathy induced by rapid ventricular pacing in dogs. *Lab Invest* 73: 771–787.

Long X, Boluyt MO, de Lourdes Hipolito M, Lundberg MS, Zheng JS, O'Neill L, Cirie lli X, Laka tta EG, Crow MT (1997). p53 and the hypoxia-induced apoptosis of cultured neonatal rat cardiac myocytes. *J Clin Invest* 99: 2635–2643.

Lowes BD, Minobe W, Abraham WT, Rizeq MN, Bohlmmeyer TJ, Quaife RA, Roden RL, Dutcher DL, Robertson AD, Voelkel NF, Badesch DB, Groves BM, Gibert ED, Bristow MR (1997). Changes in gene expression in the intact human heart. Downregulation of α–myosin heavy chain in hypertrophied, failing ventricular myocardium. *J Clin Invest* 100: 2315–2324.

Luciani M, Rocco M, Pizzolitto S, Antoci B (1991). Does the analysis of DNA in myocytes have meaning? *Pathologica* 83: 289–294.

MacLellan WR, Schneider MD (1997). Death by design. Programmed cell death in cardiovascular biology and disease. *Circ Res* 81: 137–144.

Mallat Z, Tedgui A, Fontaliran F, Frank R, Durigon M, Fontaine G (1996). Evidence of apoptosis in arrhythmogenic right ventricular dysplasia. *N Engl J Med* 335: 1190–1196.

Marchevsky A, Tolmachoff T, Lee S (1996). Quality assurance issues in DNA image cytometry. *Cytometry* 26: 101–107.

Marino TA, Haldar S, Williamson EC Beaverson K, Walter RA, Marino DR, Beatly C, Lipson KE (1991). Proliferating cell nuclear antigen in developing and adult rat cardiac muscle cells. *Circ. Res* 69: 1353–1360.

Martynova MG, Antipanova EM, Rumiantsev PP (1983). Quantity of DNA, sex chromatin bodies and nucleoli in the nuclei of the muscle cells of normal and hypertrophied human atria. *Tsitologiia* 25: 614–619.

Martynova MG, Selivanova GV, Vlasova TD (2002). Ploidy levels and the number of nuclei in cardiomyocytes of the lamprey and fish. *Tsitologiia* 44: 387–391.

Masri C, Chandrashekhar Y (2008). Apoptosis: a potentially reversible, meta-stable state of the heart. *Heart Fail Rev* 13: 175–179.

Matturri L, Biondo B, Grosso E, Lavezzi AM, Rossi L (1995). Morphometric and densitometric approach in hypertrophic cardiomyopathy (HCM). *Eur J Histochem* 39: 237–244.

McMahon JT, Ratliff NB (1990). Regeneration of adult human myocardium after acute heart transplant rejection. *J Heart Transplant* 9: 554–567.

McKay RG, Pfeffer MA, Pasternak RC, Markis JE, Come GC, Nakao C, Alderman JD, Ferguson JJ, Safian RD, Grossman W (1986). Left ventricular remodelling after myocardial infarction: A coronary to infarct expansion. *Circulation* 74: 693–702.

Meckert PC, Rivello HG, Vigliano C, González P, Favaloro R, Laguens R (2005). Endomitosis and polyploidization of myocardial cells in the periphery of human acute myocardial infarction. *Cardiovasc Res* 67: 116–123.

Metze K, Andrade LA (1991). Atypical stromal giant cells of cervix uteri-evidence of Schwann cell origin. *Pathol Res Pract* 187: 1031–1038.

Michel JB, Lattion AL, Salzmann JL Cerol ML, Philippe M, Camilleri JP, Corvol P (1988). Hormonal and cardiac effects of converting enzyme inhibition in rat myocardial infarction. *Circ Res* 62: 641–650.

Munck-Wikland E, Rubio CA, Auer GU, Kuylenstierna R, Lindholm J (1990). Control cells for image cytometric DNA analysis of esophageal tissue and the influence of preoperative treatment. *Analyt Quant Cytol Histol* 12: 267–274.

Murat JC, Gamet L, Cazenave Y, Trocheris V (1990). Questions about the use of ^{3}H thymidine incorporation as a reliable method to estimate cell proliferation rate. *Biochem J* 270: 563–564.

Nadal-Ginard B, Mahdavi (1989). Molecular basis of cardiac performance. Plasticity of the myocardium generated through protein isoform switches. *J Clin Invest* 84: 1693–1700.

Nagl W (1990). Polyploidy in differentiation and evolution. *Cell Cloning* 8: 216–223.

Nakao K, Minobe W, Roden R, Bristow MR, Leinwand LA (1997). Myosin heavy chain gene expression in human heart failure. *J Clin Invest* 100: 2362–2370.

Narula J, Haider N, Virmani R, DiSalvo TG, Kolodgie FD, Hajjar RJ, Schmidt U, Semigran MJ, Dec GW, Khaw BA (1996). Apoptosis in myocytes in end-stage heart failure. *N Engl J Med* 335:1182–1189.

Nelson-Rees WA, Kniazeff AJ, Darby NB (1966). Chromatin bridges and origin of multinucleate cells in a bovine testicular cell line. *Cytogenetics* 5: 164–178.

Nichtova Z, Novotova M, Kralova E, Stankovicova T (2012). Morphological and functional characteristics of models of experimental myocardial injury induced by isoproterenol. *Gen Physiol Biophys* 31: 141–151.

Nicol L, Jeppesen PGN (1994). Human autoimmune sera recognize a conserved protein that is homologous to *Drosophila* HP1 and is associated with mammalian heterochromatin. *Chrom Res* 2. 245–253.

Nishida K, Otsu K (2008). Cell death in heart failure. *Circ J*. 72 Suppl A: A17–A21.

Nozyński J, Zakliczyński M, Zembala-Nozyńska E, Konecka-Mrówká D, Przybylski R, Nikiel B, Mlynarczyk-Liszka J, Lange D, Mrówka A, Przybylski J, Maruszewski M, Zembala M (2009). Cardiocyte nuclear chromatin density correlates with transplanted heart left ventricular mass. *Transplant Proc.* 41: 281–287.

Oberpriller JO, Ferrans VJ, Carroll RJ (1983). Changes in DNA content, number of nuclei and cellular dimensions of young rat atrial myocytes in response to left coronary artery ligation. *J Mol Cell Cardiol* 15: 31–42.

Oberpriller JO, Oberpriller JC, Arefyeva AM, Mitashov VI, Carlson BM (1988). Nuclear characteristics of cardiac myocytes following the proliferative response to mincing of the myocardium in the adult newt, Notophthalmus viridescens. *Cell Tissue Res* 253: 619–624.

Ohara T, Little WC (2010). Evolving focus on diastolic dysfunction in patients with coronary artery disease. *Curr Opin Cardiol* 25: 613–621.

Olivero OA, Poirier MC (1993). Preferential incorporation of 3'-azido-2',3'-dideoxythymidine into telomeric DNA and Z-DNA-containing regions of Chinese hamster ovary cells. *Mol Carcinog* 8: 81–88.

Olivetti G, Abbi R, Quaini F, Kajstura J, Cheng W, Nitahara JA, Quaini E, Di Loreto C, Beltrami CA, Krajewski S, Reed JC, Anversa P (1997). Apoptosis in the failing human heart. *N Engl J Med* 336: 1131–1141.

Olivetti G, Capasso JM, Sonnenblick EH Anversa P (1990). Side-to-side slippage of myocytes participates in ventricular wall remodelling acutely after myocardial infarction in rats. *Circ Res* 67: 23–34.

Olivetti G, Cigola E, Maestri R, Corradi D, Lagrasta C, Gambert SR, Anversa P (1996a). Aging, cardiac hypertrophy and ischemic cardiomyopathy do not affect the proportion of mononucleated and multinucleated myocytes in human hearts. *J Mol Cell Cardiol* 28: 1463–1477.

Olivetti G, Melissari M, Balbi T, Quaini F, Cigola E, Sonnenblick EH, Anversa P (1994a). Myocyte cellular hypertrophy is responsible for ventricilar remodelling in the hypertrophied heart of middle aged individuals in the absence of cardiac failure. *Cardiovasc Res* 28: 1199–1208.

Olivetti G, Melissari M, Balbi T, Quaini F, Sonnenblick EH, Anversa P (1994b). Myocyte nuclear and possible cellular hyperplasia contribute to ventricular remodeling in the hypertrophic senescent heart in humans. *J Am Cell Cardiol* 24: 140–149.

Olivetti G, Melissari M, Capasso JM, Anversa P (1991). Cardiomyopathy of the aging human heart: myocyte loss and reactive cellular hypertrophy. *Circ. Rec* 68: 1560–1568.

Olivetti G, Quaini F, Sala R, Lagrasta C, Corradi D, Bonacina E, Gambert SR, Cigola E, Anversa P (1996b). Acute myocardial infarction in humans is associated with activation of programmed myocyte cell death in the surviving portion of the heart. *J Mol Cell Cardiol* 28: 2005–2016.

Olivetti G, Ricci R, Anversa P (1987). Hyperplasia of myocyte nuclei in long-term cardiac hypertrophy in rats. *J Clin Invest* 80: 1818–1822

Olivetti G, Ricci R, Lagrasta C, Maniga E, Sonnenblick EH, Anversa P (1988). Cellular basis of wall remodeling in long-term pressure overload-induced right ventricular hypertrophy in rats. *Circ Res* 63: 648–657.

Olson TM (2006). What makes the heart fail? New insights from defective genes. *Acta Paediatr Suppl.* 95: 17–21.

O'Sullivan JN, Bronner MP, Brentnall TA, Finley JC, Shen WT, Emerson S, Emond MJ, Gollahon KA, Moskovitz AH, Crispin DA, Potter JD, Rabinovitch PS (2002). Chromosomal instability in ulcerative colitis is related to telomere shortening. *Nat Genet* 32: 280–284.

Page E (1978). Quantitative ultrastructureal analysis in cardiac membrane physiology. *Am J Physiol* 235: C147–C158.

Panizo-Santos A, Sola JJ, Pardo-Mindan FJ, Hernandez M, Cenarruzabeitia E, Diez J (1995). Angiotensin converting enzyme inhibition prevents polyploidization of cardiomyocytes in spontaneously hypertensive rats with left ventricular hypertrophy. *J Pathol* 431–437.

Pantely GA, Bristow JD (1984). Ischemic cardiomyopathy. *Prog Cardiovasc Dis* 27: 95–114.

Parker TG, Schneider MD (1991). Growth factors, proto-oncogenes, and plasticity of the cardiac phenotype. *Annu Rev Physiol* 53: 179–200.

Parodi O, De Maria R, Oltrona L, Testa R, Sambuceti G, Roghi A, Merli M, Belingheri L, Accinni R Spinelli F, Pellegrini A, Baroldi G (1993). Myocardial blood flow distribution in patients with ischemic heart disease or dilated cardiomyopathy undergoing heart transplantation. *Circulation* 88: 509–522.

Pepper JR, Khagani A, Yacoub M (1995). Heart transplantation. *J Antimicr Chem* 36, Suppl: 23–38.

Petrashchuk OM, Oniskchenko GE (1987). Role of multipolar mitoses in the proliferation of multinucleate cells induced by cytochalasin B. *Tsitologiia* 29: 794–801.

Pfeffer MA, Braunwald E (1990). Ventricular remodeling after myocardial infarction. *Circulation* 81: 1161–1172.

Pomerance A, Stovin P (1985) Heart transplant pathology: the British experience. *J Clin Pathol* 38: 146–159.

Prasher N, Prasher BS (1989). Congenital dyserythropoietic anaemia. *J Assoc Physicians India* 37: 467–468.

Quaini F, Cigola E, Lagrasta C, Saccani G, Quaini E, Rossi C, Olivetti G, Anversa P (1994). End-stage cardiac failure in humans is coupled with the induction of proliferating cell nuclear antigen and nuclear mitotic division in ventricular myocytes. *Circ Res* 75: 1050–1063.

Rakusan K (1984). Cardiac growth, maturation and aging. In Zak R (ed): *Growth of the Heart in Health and Disease*. New York, Raven Press Publishers, pp 131–164.

Rakusan K, Flanagan MF, Geva T, Southern J, Van Praagh R (1992). Morphometry of human coronary capilaries during normal growth and the effect of age in left ventricular pressure-overload hypertrophy. *Circulation* 86: 38–46.

Rakusan K, Korecky B (1985). Regression of cardiomegaly induced in newborn rats. *Can J Cardiol* 1: 217–222.

Reasor MJ, Massey CA, Koshut RA, Castranova V (1982). Multinucleation in alveolar macrophages from rats treated with chlorphentermine. *Lab Invest* 46: 224–230.

Reiss K, Kjstura J, Capasso JM, Marino TA, Anversa P (1993). Impairment of myocyte contractility following coronary artery narrowing is associated with activation of the myocyte IGF-1 autocrine system, enhanced expression of late growth related genes, DNA synthesis and myocyte nuclear mitotic division in rats. *Exp Cell Res* 207: 348–360.

Reiss K, Kajstura J, Zhang X, Li P, Szoke K, Olivetti G, Anversa P (1994). Acute myocardial infarction leads to up-regulation of the IGF-1 autocrine system, DNA replication, and nuclear mitotic division in the remaining viable cardiac myocytes. *Exp Cell Res* 213: 463–472.

Rizzoni M, Cundari E, Perticone P, Gustavino B (1993). Chromatin bridges between sister chromatids induced in late G2 mitosis in CHO cells by trimethylpsoralen + UVA. *Exp Cell Res* 209: 149–155.

Rivello HG, Meckert PC, Vigliano C, Favaloro R, Laguens RP (2001). Cardiac myocyte nuclear size and ploidy status decrease after mechanical support. *Cardiovasc Pathol* 10: 53–57.

Roberts WC (1976). The coronary arteries and left ventricle in clinically isolated angina pertoris: A necropsy analysis. *Circulation* 54: 388–390.

Rosenberg B, Pfitzer P (1983). Ploidy in the hearts of elderly patients. *Virchows Arch (Cell Pathol)* 42: 19–24.

Rowan RA, Billingham ME (1990). Pathological changes in the long-term transplanted hearts. A morphometric study of myocardial hypertrophy, vascularity and fibrosis. *Hum Pathol* 21: 767–772.

Rumyantsev PP (1965). DNA synthesis and nuclear division in embryonal and postnatal histogenesis of myocardium (autoradiographic study). *Fef Ptoc* 24: 899–902.

Rumyantsev PP, Erokhina IL, Antipanova EM, Martynova MG (1990). DNA and sex chromatin centent in nuclei of conductive system and working myocytes of normal and hypertrophied human heart. *Acta Histochem Suppl* 39: 225–237.

Rumyantsev PP, Kassem AM (1976). Cumulative indices of DNA synthesizing myocytes in different compartments of the working myocardium and conductive system of the rat heart muscle following extensive left ventricular infarction. *Virchows Arch B Cell Pathol* 20: 329–342.

Sandritter W, Scomazzoni G (1964). Deoxyribonucleic acid content (Feulgen photometry) and dry weight (interference microscopy) of normal and hypertrophic heart muscle fibers. *Nature (Lond.)* 202: 100–101.

Sansone G, Lupi L (1991). An aberrant type of congenital dyserythropoietic anemia associated with a beta-thalassemia trait. *Ann Hematol* 62: 184–187.

Sato S, Burgess SB, McIlwain DL (1994). Transcription and motoneuron size. *J Neurochem* 63: 1609–1615.

Saunders WS, Chue C, Goebl M, Craig C, Clark RF, Powers JA, Eissenberg JC, Elgin SCR, Rothfield NF, Earnshaw WC (1993). Molecular cloning of a human homologue of *Drosophila* heterochromatin protein HP1 using anti-centrome autoantibodies with anti-chromo specificity. *J Cell Sci* 104: 573–582.

Savinova OV, Gerdes AM (2012). Myocyte changes in heart failure. *Heart Fail Clin* 8: 1–6.

Schaper J, Froede R, Hein S, Buck A, Hashizume H, Speiser B, Friedl A, Bleese N (1991). Impairment of myocardial ultrastructure and changes of the cytoskeleton in dilated cardiomyopathy. *Circilation* 83: 504–514.

Schmid G, Pfitzer P (1985). Mitoses and binucleated cells in perinatal human hearts. *Virchows Arch B Cell Pathol Incl Mol Pathol* 48: 59–67.

Scheneider MD, Payne PA, Ueno H, Perryman MB, Roberto R (1986). Dissociated expression of e-myc and a fos-related competence gene during cardiac myogenesis. *Mol Cell Biol* 6: 4140–4143.

Schuster EH, Bulkley BH (1980). Ischemic cardiomyopathy: A clinicopathologic study of fourteen patients. *Am Heart J* 100: 506–512.

Sharov VG, Sabbah HN, Shimoyama H, Goussev AV, Lesch M, Goldstein S (1996). Evidence of cardiocyte apoptosis in myocardium of dogs with chronic heart failure. *Am J Pathol* 148: 141–149.

Shperling ID, Mirakian VO, Petrosian DG (1983). Characteristics of isolated cardiomyocytes of the left regions of the human heart in hypertrophy. *Arkh Patol* 45: 52–55.

Simpson PC (1989). Proto-oncogenes and cardiac hypertrophy. *Annu Res Physiol* 51: 189–202.

Skalli O, Gabbiani G, Babai F, Seemayer TA, Pizzolato G, Schurch W (1988). Intermediate filament protein and actin isoforms as markers for soft tissue tumor differentiation and origin. II. Rhabdomyosarcomas. *Am J Pathol* 130: 515–531.

Smith MJ, Ortaldo JR (1993). Mechanisms of cytotoxicity used by human peripheral blood CD4+ and CD8+ T cell subsets: the role of franule exocytosis. *J Immunol* 151: 740–747.

Starr DA, Williams BC, Li Z, Etemad-Moghadam B, Dawe RK, Goldberg ML (1997). Conservation of the centromere/kinetochore protein ZW10. *J Cell Biol* 138: 1289–1301.

Suitters AJ, Rose ML, Dominguez MY, Yacoub MH (1990). Selection of donor specific cytotoxic lymphocytes within the allografted human heart. *Transplantation* 49: 105–110.

Symmans WF, Nielsen H, Dell R, Rose E, Marboe CC (1994). Cardiac allograft pathology: a clinicopathologic correlation. *Cardiovasc Pathol* 3: 249–256.

Szabolcs M, Michler RE, Yang XC, Aji W, Roy D, Athan E, Sciacca RR, Minanov OP, Cannon PJ (1996). Apoptosis of cardiac myocytes during cardiac allograft rejection. Relation to the induction of nitric oxide synthase. *Circulation* 94: 1665–1673.

Takamatsu T, Nakanishi K, Fukuda M, Fujita S (1983). Cytofluorometric nuclear DNA-determinations in infant, adolescent, adult and aging human hearts. *Histochemistry* 77: 485–494.

Takeda K, Yu Z, Nishikawa T, Tanaka M, Hosoda S, Ferrans VJ, Kasajima T (1996). Apoptosis and DNA fragmentation in the bulbus cordis of the developing heart. *J Mol Cell Cardiol* 28: 209–215.

Takubo T, Kitano K, Ikemoto T, Kikuchi T, Shimizu A (1993). Ring eosinophils in patients with lowered eosinophil peroxidase activity. *Rinsho Byori* 41: 468–470.

Tanaka M, Ito H, Adachi S, Akimoto H, Nishikawa T, Kasajima T, Marimo F, Hiroe M (1994). Hypoxia induces apoptosis with enhanced expression of fax antigen messenger RNA in cultured neonatal rat cardiomyocytes. *Circ Res* 75: 426–433.

Tate JM, Oberpriller JO, Oberpriller JC (1989). Analysis of DNA synthesis in cell cultures of the adult newt cardiac myocyte. *Tissue Cell* 21: 335–342.

Tazelaar HD, Edwands WD (1992). Pathology of cardiac transplantation: recipient hearts (chronic heart failure) and donor hearts (acute and chronic rejection). *Mayo Clin Proc* 67: 685–696.

Teiger E, Dam TV, Richard L, Wisnewsky C, Tea BS, Gaboury L, Tremblay J, Schwartz K, Hamet P (1996). Apoptosis in pressure overload induced heart hypertrophy in the rat. *J Clin Invest* 97: 2891–2897.

Tekola P, Baak JPA, Belien JAM, Brugghe J (1994). Highly sensitive, specific, and stable new fluorescent DNA stains for confocal laser microscopy and image processing of normal paraffin sections. *Cytometry* 17: 191–195.

Tournamille J, Caporiccio B, Michel R, Sentein P (1982). Effect of methylmercury chloride on mitosis in human lymphocytes in culture: ultrastructural study. *C R Seances Soc Biol Fil* 176: 194–203.

Tusell L, Pampalona J, Soler D, Frías C, Genescà A (2010). Different outcomes of telomere-dependent anaphase bridges. *Biochem Soc Trans* 38: 1698–1703.

Ueno H, Perryman MB, Roberts R, Schneider MD (1988). Differentiation of cardiac myocytes after mitogen withdrawal exihibits three sequential states of the ventricular growth response. *J Cell Biol* 107: 1911–1918.

Unverferth DV, Baker PB, Swift SE Chaffee R, Fetters JK, Uretsky BF, Thompson ME, Leier CV (1986). Extent of myocardial fibrosis and cellular hypertrophy in dilated cardiomyopathy. *Am J Cardiol* 57: 816–820.

Urbanek K, Torella D, Sheikh F, De Angelis A, Nurzynska D, Silvestri F, Beltrami CA, Bussani R, Beltrami AP, Quaini F, Bolli R, Leri A, Kajstura J, Anversa P (2005). Myocardial regeneration by activation of multipotent cardiac stem cells in ischemic heart failure. *Proc Natl Acad Sci USA* 102: 8692–8697.

van der Laarse A, Bloys van Treslong CH, Vliegen HW, Ricciardi L (1987). Relation between ventricular DNA content and number of myocytes and non-myocytes in hearts of normotensive and spontaneously hypertensive rats. *Cardiovasc Res* 21: 223–229.

van der Laarse A, Hollaar L, Vliegen HW, Egas JM, Dijkshoorn NJ, Cornelisse CJ, Bogers AJ, Quaegebeur JM (1989a). Myocardial (iso) enzyme activities, DNA concentration and nuclear polyploidy in hearts of patients operated upon for congenital heart disease, and in normal and hypertrophic adult human hearts at autopsy. *Eur J Clin Invest* 19: 192–200.

van der Laarse A, Vliegen HW, van der Nat KH, Hollaar L, Egas JM, Swier GP, van den Broek AJ (1989b). Comparison of myocardial changes between pressure induced hypertrophy and normal growth in the rat heart. *Cardiovasc Res* 23: 308–314.

van Kesteren CA, van Heugten HA, Lamers JM, Saxena PR, Schalekamp MA, Danser AH (1997). Angiotensin II-mediated growth and antigrowth effects in cultured neonatal rat cardiac myocytes and fibroblasts. *J Mol Cell Cardiol* 29: 2147–2157.

van Suylenet RJ, van Bekkum EEC, Boersma H, de Kok LB, Baik AHMM, Bos E, Bosman FT (1996). Collagen content and distribution in the normal and transplanted human heart: A postmortem quantitative light microscopic analysis. *Cardiovasc Pathol* 5: 61–68.

Vasil'eva IA, Aref'eva AM (1988). The ratio in the DNA content and protein mass of human cardiomyocytes. *Biull Eksp Biol Med* 106: 227–229.

Verbunt RJ, den Ottolander GJ, Kluin PM, Brederoo P, Kluin-Nelemans HC (1989). Circulating buttock cells in non-Hodgkin's lymphoma. *Leukemia* 3: 578–584.

Vliegen HW, Bruschke AV, van der Lassrse A (1990). Different responses of cellular DNA content to cardiac hypertrophy in human and rat heart myocytes. *Comp Biochem Physiol A* 95: 109–114.

Vliegen HW, van der Laarse A, Cornelisse CJ, Eulderink F (1991). Myocardial changes in pressure overload-induced left ventricular hypertrophy. A study on tissue composition, polyploidization and multinucleation. *Eur Heart J* 12: 488–494.

Vliegen HW, van der Laarse A, Huysman JA, Wijnvoord EC, Mentar M, Cornelisse CJ, Enlderink F (1987). Morphometric quantification of myocyte dimensions validated in normal growing rat hearts and applied to hypertrophic human hearts. *Cardiovasc Res* 21: 352–357.

Vliegen HW, Vossepoel AM, van der Laarse A, Cornelisse CJ (1986). Methodological aspects of flow cytometry analysis of DNA polypolidy in human heart tissue. *Histochemistry* 84: 348–353.

Voldes PGA, Willems IEMG, Cleutjens JPM, Arends JW, Havenith MG, Daemen MJAP (1993). Interstitial collagen is increased in the non-infarcted human myocardium after myocardial infarction. *J Mol Cell Cardiol* 25: 1317–1323.

Wagner M, Siddiqui MA (2009). Signaling networks regulating cardiac myocyte survival and death. *Curr Opin Investig Drugs* 10: 928–937.

Warnes CA, Roberts WC (1984). Sudden coronary death: Relation of amount and distribution of coronary narrowing at necropsy to previous symptoms of myocardial ischemia, left ventricular scarring and heart weight. *Am J Cardiol* 54: 65–73.

Warren SE, Royald HD, Markis JE, Grossman W, McKay RG (1988). Time course of left ventricular dilation after myocardial infarction: Influence of infarct-related artery and success of coronary thrombolysis. *J Am Coll Cardiol* 11: 12–19.

White WL, Zhang YL, Shelby J Trautman MS, Perkins SL, Hammond EH, Shaddy RE (1997). Myocardial apoptosis in a heterotopic murine heart transplantation model of chronic rejection and graft vasculopathy. *J Heart Lung Transplant* 16: 250–255.

Winters GL (1991). The pathology of heart allograft rejection. *Arch Pathol Lab Med* 115: 266–272.

Wolf KW, Mentzel M, Mndoza AS (1996). DNA-containing cytoplasmic bridges in a human breast cancer cell line, MX-1: morphological markers of a highly mobile cell type? *J Submicrosc Cytol Pathol* 28: 369–373.

Wreggett KA, Hill F, James PS, Hutchings A, Butcher GW, Singh PB (1994). A mammalian homologue of *Drosophila* heterochromatin protein 1 (HP1) is a component of constitutive heterochromatin. *Cytogenet Cell Genet* 66: 99–103.

Yan SM, Finato N, Artico D, Di Loreto C, Cataldi P, Bussani R, Silvesti F, Beltrami CA (1998). DNA content, apoptosis and mitosis in transplanted human hearts. *Adv Clin Path* 2: 205–219.

Yan SM, Finato N, Di Loreto C, Beltrami CA (1999a). Nuclear size of myocardial cells in end-stage cardiomyopathies. *Analyt Quant Cytol Histol* 21: 174–180.

Yan SM, Guerra S, Finato N, Di Loreto C, Beltrami CA (1999b). Changes in DNA content of myocardial cells after cardiac explantation. *Adv Clin Path* 3: 23–27.

Zerbini C, Weinberg DS, Perez-Atayde AR (1992). DNA ploidy analysis of myocardial hyperplasia. *Hum Pathol* 23: 1427–1430.

Zimmerman W, Sparks CA, Doxsey SJ (1999). Amorphous no longer: the centrosome comes into focus. *Curr Opin Cell Biol* 11: 122–128.

8. ABBREVIATIONS

AVONA	one-way analysis of variance
AZT	3'-azido-2',3'-dideoxythymidine
BFB	breakage-fusion-bridge
CKAP2	cytoskeleton associated protein 2
CV	coefficient of variation
CVANA	the coefficient of variation in average nuclear area
CHO	Chinese hamster ovary
DDW	double distilled water
DI	DNA index
hCSCs	human cardiac stem cells
IOD	integrated optical density
KOH	potassium hydroxide
MP	mean ploidy
NYHA	New York Heart Association
PCNA	proliferating cell nuclear antigen
PICH	Plk1-interacting checkpoint helicase
PF	polyploidization factor
SCCBs	sister chromatid chromatin bridges
SD	standard deviation
SPP	sum of ploidy peaks
SIP	sum of intermediate ploidies
TPI	total ploidy index
TMP	trimethylpsoralen
TMAP	tumor-associated microtubule-associated protein
TRITC	tetra-methyl-rhodamine isothiocyanate
UVA	ultraviolet type A

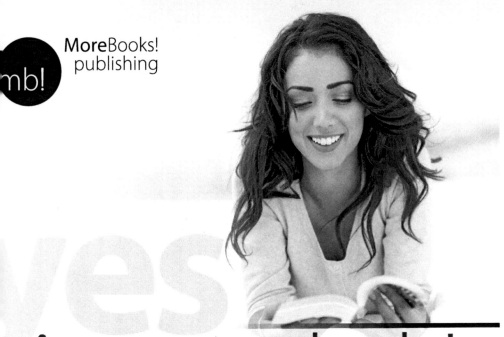

Lightning Source UK Ltd.
Milton Keynes UK
UKOW04f0855180913

217436UK00001B/205/P